Childbirth-Related Pelvic Floor Dysfunction

Diego Riva • Gianfranco Minini
Editors

Childbirth-Related Pelvic Floor Dysfunction

Risk Factors, Prevention, Evaluation, and Treatment

Springer

Editors
Diego Riva
Department of Gynecology
"S. Pio X" Clinic
Milan
Italy

Gianfranco Minini
Urogynecology
"Città di Brescia" Clinic Institute
Brescia
Italy

ISBN 978-3-319-18196-7 ISBN 978-3-319-18197-4 (eBook)
DOI 10.1007/978-3-319-18197-4

Library of Congress Control Number: 2015949393

Springer Cham Heidelberg New York Dordrecht London

Printed on acid-free paper

Springer International Publishing AG Switzerland is part of Springer Science+Business Media
(www.springer.com)

Foreword

Perineal trauma is a common event in labour, affecting up to 90 % of primigravidas and it is sometimes associated with considerable post-natal morbidity.

Statistics show that one in ten women after vaginal delivery will have pelvic floor dysfunction, so severe that surgery may be required. All authors actually agree that the obstetric pelvic floor trauma is a heavy reality.

Even if the topic of perineal damage following delivery is widely debated in many courses and meetings, it seems very interesting having put together different specialized approaches: I believe that this text can be very useful not only for students but even for every clinician searching for a real upgrading in this field.

The strong scientific methodology and the deep analysis of the literature allow to reach a super-specialized point of view, which is necessary to look at these complex problems.

This book offers an up-to-date overview of childbirth-related pelvic floor dysfunction covering prevention, diagnosis and management. It encompasses all relevant conditions with particular focus on genital prolapse and urinary and fecal incontinence.

Risk factors for pelvic floor damage related to childbirth are identified, and a 3D simulation of delivery is presented.

The role of various diagnostic tools, including pelvic floor ultrasonography and MRI, is clearly described.

The importance of physiotherapy in preventing future alterations is explained, and the indications for surgery, which is reserved for more severe situations, are discussed.

The need for a multidisciplinary approach involving obstetricians, gynecologists, urologists, midwives, radiologists, physiotherapists, muscle laboratory engineers, and computer technicians is heavily underlined.

In conclusion, I am sure that this book represents a useful instrument to prevent and treat perineal dysfunction, contributing to female well-being, with important social and economic consequences; it will be seen with great interest from all clinicians involved in the care of female pelvic floor disorders.

Roberto Carone
President of Italian Continence Foundation
Director of Urological Unit and Spinal Lesions Center – CRF Hospital
Director of Neuro-Urological Dept M Adelaide Hosp – Turin, Italy

Preface

Recent progress in obstetrics and in midwife art deserve more attention to perineal integrity during vaginal delivery: the hands-off approach allows a more progressive distention of pelvic floor muscles and a restricted use of episiotomy can reduce the risk of perineal lesions, in comparison to the aggressive approach frequently taught in obstetric schools during the 1970s and 1980s.

Many questions regarding the best way to warrant the integrity of pelvic floor during delivery and the identification of risk factors for jeopardizing muscular lesions are yet unresolved. The relative weight of many variables such as fetal diameters or maternal weight must be taken into full account. And again: which is the more physiologic technique to perform vaginal delivery in the different normal or abnormal situations and which instruments can we use to reach a better understanding of muscle functions before and after childbearing? Can ultrasonography or magnetic resonance help us to have a full evaluation of pelvic floor integrity or of the damage? And what may we affirm about electromyography? Unfortunately we cannot yet be sure that the examinations of all these factors can allow us to reach a complete acknowledgment of the relationship between the structures of maternal pelvis and fetal body, but we cannot accept the suggestion that an extensive use of cesarean section could eliminate these problems, as many data coming from recent literature speak against this point of view.

As a matter of fact we believe that modern obstetrics cannot know a complete progress without a deep understanding of all factors implied in the wonderful and for many aspects unresolved mechanism of delivery, but we must work with nature to minimize and possibly prevent the damage.

The purpose of this text is to help all practitioners, thanks to its multidisciplinary approach, to walk along the field of diagnosis and treatment of pelvic floor dysfunction related to delivery, in an attempt to allow to our pregnant patients to go through their childbearing without the fear of the dangerous consequences of permanent muscle lesions.

This challenge is before us, and it is time to work again along this road.

Therefore, we must surely and sincerely thank all the fantastic colleagues who accepted to help us to complete this text.

Our thanks and our remembrance go also to our great friend Lorenzo Spreafico, who left us 2 years ago, after having showed us during his life a great attention to patients during their pregnancies and deliveries, and a full ability in the field of pelvic floor surgery.

At the end, but not least, a great thanks to our wives and to our families who supported us during this work.

Milan, Italy Diego Riva
Brescia, Italy Gianfranco Minini

Contents

1 Anatomy and Physiology of the Pelvic Floor 1
Gianni F.A. Baudino

2 Perineal and Anal Sphincter Obstetric Injury 25
Gianfranco Minini

3 A Computerized Model of Pelvic Floor Muscles Physiology During Delivery 35
Maurizio Serati and Giorgio Bogani

4 Clinical Approach to the Evaluation of Pelvic Floor Dysfunctions 41
Giancarlo Vignoli

5 Echographic Diagnosis of Childbirth-Related Pelvic Floor Injuries 51
Giulio A. Santoro and Maher A. Abbas

6 Combined Three-Dimensional Transperineal Ultrasonography (3-D TPUS) and Magnetic Resonance Imaging (MRI) After Vaginal Delivery 69
Vittorio L. Piloni and Fabio Muggia

7 Pelvic Floor EMG: Principles, Techniques, and Applications 83
Roberto Merletti

8 Sexual Function After Delivery 101
Stefano Salvatore, Anna Redaelli, Ilaria Baini, and Massimo Candiani

9 The Controversial Role of Episiotomy 105
Diego Riva

10 Perineal Care During Pregnancy, Delivery, and Postpartum 115
Giuseppe Ettore, Gabriella Torrisi, and Sebastiana Ferraro

11 Genital Prolapse and Urinary Incontinence After Childbirth 135
Francesco Marson and Luisella Squintone

12 Fecal Incontinence After Childbirth: Diagnostic and Clinical Aspects 143
Alvise Frasson and Giuseppe Dodi

13 Principles and Methods of Physiotherapy After Delivery 155
Simonetta Minoli

14 Surgery for Urinary Incontinence and Prolapse Shortly After Childbirth 165
Luisa Ricci

15 A Practical Approach to Pelvic Floor Dysfunctions After Childbirth: Diagnostic and Therapeutic Flowcharts 171
Antonella Biroli

16 Clinical Cases 185
Arianna Bortolami

Index 195

Anatomy and Physiology of the Pelvic Floor

1

Gianni F.A. Baudino

1.1 Introduction: The Pelvic Content

The small pelvis in the female contains three reservoirs made of smooth muscle, an inner mucosal layer and a fibro-adipose adventitia externally. The bundles running together with the hypogastric fascia, from the pelvic sidewalls toward the midline, provide blood and nerve supply. The bladder is a true reservoir, since it is closed upward by the vesico-ureteral valves and downward by the urethral smooth- and rhabdosphincter. The vagina is not a proper reservoir, since it has not any biologic fluid or solid to contain, but it is the site of the dramatic accommodation that takes place during childbirth. It communicates upward with the cervix, which is part of the birth canal and has an open bottom that is the introitus. The vagina has not a real sphincter at its introitus, but the perineal membrane and muscles, together with the perineal body can be seen as a closure mechanism. Posteriorly the rectum is a particular kind of reservoir with slow transit, open top and a complex sphincteric system. All the three viscera have a proper morphology, a definite relationship one to each other, and a typical position inside the pelvis. These features are strictly associated with their function, as for storage and emptying phases. The position and mobility of each organ is basically provided by two mechanisms: On one hand the fixation systems to the connective and muscular structures of the pelvis, which are real mesenteries and act as ligaments holding the viscera in place and, on the other hand, the pelvic floor muscles that support the pelvic content, close the genital hiatus and compensate the abdominal rising pressures. In particular the

G.F.A. Baudino
Azienda Ospedaliera Ospedale Maggiore di Crema, Largo Ugo Dossena n.2, Crema 26013, Italy
e-mail: baudino03@gmail.com

D. Riva, G. Minini (eds.), *Childbirth-Related Pelvic Floor Dysfunction: Risk Factors, Prevention, Evaluation, and Treatment*,
DOI 10.1007/978-3-319-18197-4_1

muscular sling of the pubococcygeus lifts and moves upward and forward the whole pelvic content, acting as an additional sphincter. The pelvic floor is a dynamic unit that allows the physiology of continence, emptying, sexual function and delivery. Pelvic ligaments and fasciae are the anatomic connections that allow viscera and muscles to work together.

The ligaments of the pelvic regions are usually considered by most anatomists as parts of the thickened retropelvic fascia that run along blood and lymphatic vessels, nerves and connective tissue, while surgeons consider it as a true fascial layer. It becomes denser adjacent to the lateral aspects of uterine cervix and vagina, being usually called broad ligament; it is formed by a thin, double plication of the peritoneum connecting the lateral pelvic structures to the uterus. The corresponding fascia that links the cervix and the vagina to the pelvic wall is called cardinal or Mackenrodt's ligament. The posterior part of this fascia extending from the upper portion of the cervix to the sacral vertebra are indicated as uterosacral ligaments.

1.2 The Bony Pelvis

It is made of the two symmetrical coxal or hip bones (composed of ileum, ischium, and pubis), sacrum and coccyx. The hip bones are fused to the sacrum posteriorly and to each other anteriorly at the pubic symphysis.

The bony pelvis is divided into superior or false or greater pelvis and inferior or true or smaller pelvis by the pelvic brim, whose structures are the sacral promontory, the anterior sacral ala, the arcuate line of the ilium, the pectineal pubic line and the pubic crest that ends in the pubic symphysis.

The inferior pelvic outlet is closed by the pelvic floor. The muscles of this regions have two fundamental functions: they provide support or act as a "floor" for the abdominal viscera including the rectum, and constrictor or continence mechanism to the urethral, anal, and vaginal orifices (in females).

In comparison to males, females have a pelvis with wider diameter and a more circular shape (Fig. 1.1). The wider inlet facilitates the engagement of the fetal head and parturition. On the other hand, this shape predisposes to subsequent pelvic floor weakness. Attachment sites for ligaments, muscles, and fascial layers are provided by a number of projections and contours.

The ischial spine, at the midst of the brim of the ischiatic foramen, is the anchorage of several connective and muscular tissues. Some authors describe the spine and the related ligament complex as a star. The sacrospinous ligament, the coccygeal muscle, the posterior portion of the arcus tendineus fasciae pelvis, and the arcus tendineus levator ani leaving the spine stand like beams around it. The sacrospinous ligament extends from the ischial spines to the lateral margins of the sacrum and coccyx anteriorly to the sacrotuberous ligament. During the dissection it can be seen as a separate structure, just behind the ischiococcigeus muscle, or as a complex with the muscle, superficial or deep. The greater and lesser sciatic foramina are above and below the ligament (Fig. 1.2).

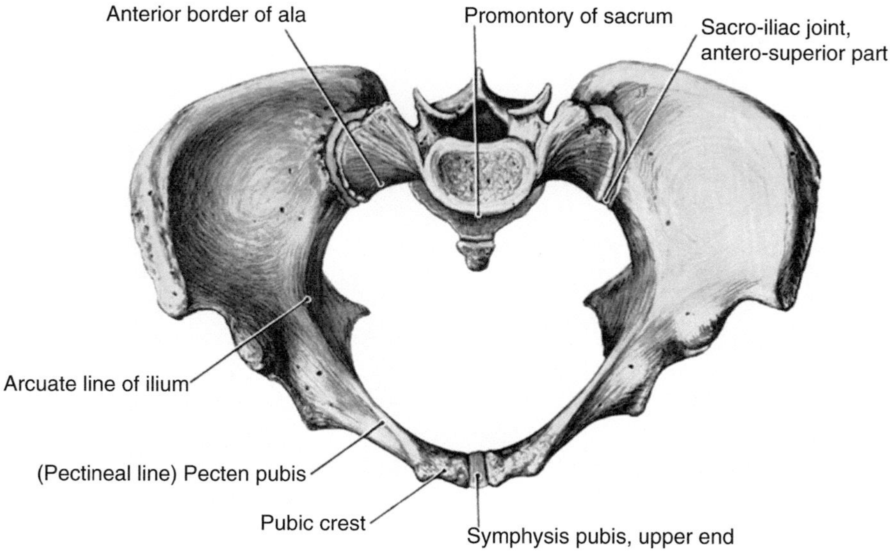

Fig. 1.1 The female bony pelvis

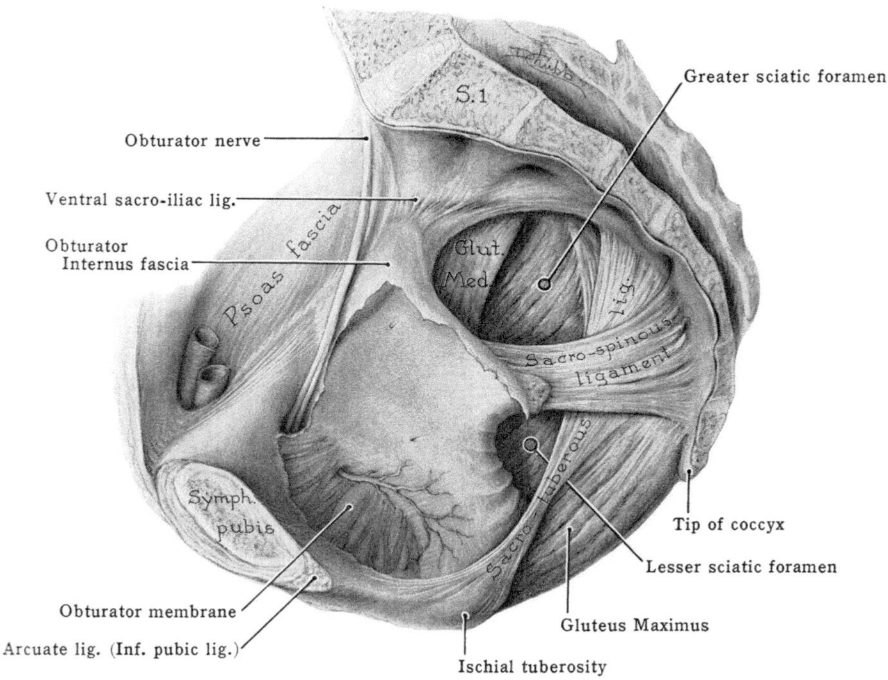

Fig. 1.2 The female bony pelvis with the sacro-spinous and the sacro-tuberous ligaments ant the greater and lesser sciatic foramen (Grant (1962) An atlas of anatomy)

1.3 The Muscular Pelvic Floor

1.3.1 Pelvic Diaphragm

The pelvic diaphragm is a thin and wide muscular structure that forms the inferior limit of the abdominopelvic cavity. It is formed of a tunnel-shaped muscle that extends with its fascia from the symphysis pubis to the coccyx and laterally from one wall of the pelvis to the other. The levator ani and coccygeus muscles that are attached to the internal surface of the minor pelvis form the muscular floor of the pelvis.

They originate from the pubic bone at the level of pectinate line and from the obturator internus fascia and are connected to the coccyx.

The levator ani muscle (LAM) is composed of two major muscles: the pubococcygeus and iliococcygeus muscles from medial to lateral. The medial portion of the LA is the bulky pubococcygeus muscle that takes origin from the middle of inferior pubic rami, the pubic symphysis and anterior portion of its arcus tendineus. The arcus tendineus of the LA is indeed a dense structure made of connective tissue, running from the pubic ramus to the ischial spine along the surface of the obturator internus muscle. The muscle passes behind the rectum in an almost horizontal direction. The inner aspect forms the margin of the urogenital hiatus, which is crossed by the urethra, vagina, and anorectum.

The medial portions of the pubococcygeus has been divided in various subparts to reflect the attachments of the muscle to the urethra, vagina, anus, and rectum [1]. These portions are often called by some investigators as the pubourethralis, pubovaginalis, puboanalis, and puborectalis muscles or, all together, as the puboviscera-lis muscle, because of their attachment to the pelvic viscera [2].

The puboviscerالis definition was originally championed by Lawson and currently supported by a lot of writings of Delancey [3, 4]. While this term is well accepted in the urogynecological literature, it is rarely mentioned in the anatomical or gastroenterology textbooks.

Lawson felt that the portions of the puboviscerالis muscle are inserted into the urethra, vagina, anal canal and perineal body and he assigned respectively the names pubouretheralis, pubovaginalis, puboperinealis, and puboanalis muscles to those portions.

The urethral portion of the muscle forms part of the periurethral musculature; parallely the vaginal and anorectal parts insert into the vaginal walls, perineal body, and external anal sphincter (EAS) [5].

Posteriorly the puborectalis portion passes behind the rectal canal and is fused with the muscle of the opposite site to form a sling behind the rectum itself.

Other parts of the pubococcygeus run more posteriorly taking attachment to the coccyx.

The lateral part of the levator ani is rather thin and is called iliococcygeus; it takes origin from the arcus tendineus of the levator ani and reaches the ischial spine and the last two segments of the coccyx. The fibers from the two sides also fuse to form a raphe denominated as the anococcygeal ligament. This median raphe linking the anus and the coccyx is known as the levator plate and is the structure on which the pelvic organs rest. It is formed by the connection of the two iliococcygeus and the posterior fibers of the pubococcygeus. During the standing position, the plate is almost horizontal and supports the pelvic viscera situated just above, that is the rectum and the upper two thirds of vagina. Every event leading to a weakness of the levator ani affects this plate and may cause the levator plate to sag. As a consequence of that, the urogenital hiatus opens and predisposes to pelvic organ prolapse. Women affected by genital prolapse have been shown to have an enlarged urogenital hiatus [6, 7].

The coccygeus muscle that runs from the ischial spine to the coccyx and to the lower portion of the sacrum forms the posterior part of the pelvic diaphragm. It is situated on the anterior surface of the sacrospinous ligament (Fig. 1.3). Using 3D MRI imaging of the pelvic diaphragm, we can clearly verify its peripheral attachments and illustrate the urogenital hiatus [8].

As regards the type of these striated muscle, it has been shown that the majority of the fibers are of the slow-twitch type: they can maintain a constant tone (type I) [9] while an increased presence of fast-twitch (type II) fibers is present in the periurethral and perianal areas. This concept confirms that the normal levator ani maintains its tone in the upright position to support the pelvic viscera. Furthermore, a voluntary contraction of the puborectalis during squeezing may increase the tone to balance an increased intra-abdominal pressure.

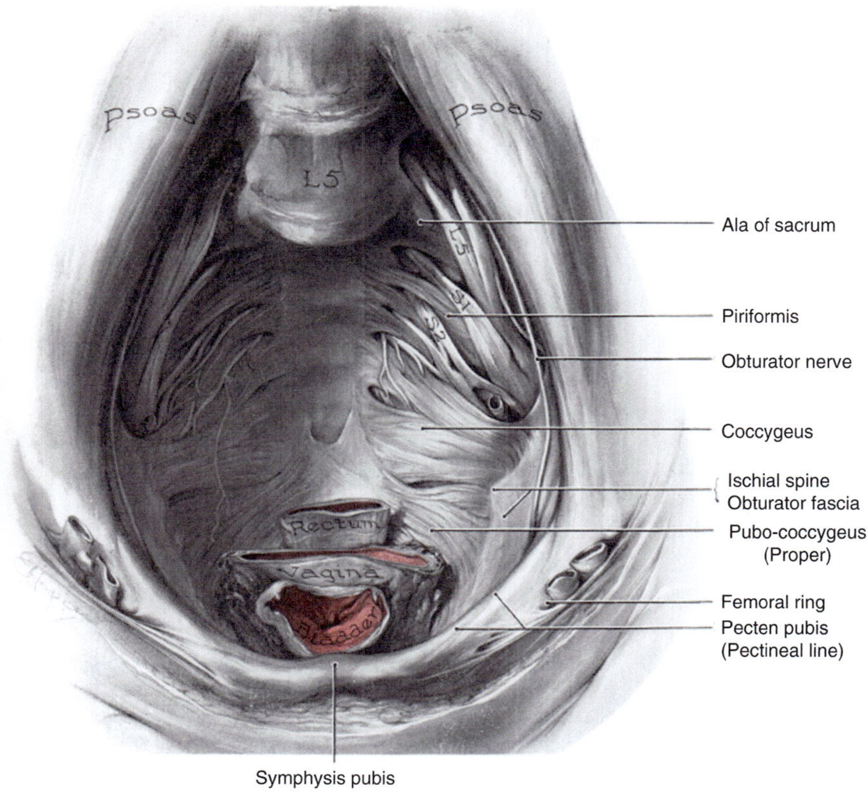

Fig. 1.3 The levator ani and its components

The urogenital diaphragm, also called the triangular ligament, is a strong, muscular membrane that lies in the area between the symphysis pubis and ischial tuberosities being therefore situated in the triangular anterior portion of the pelvic outlet.

The analysis of the urethral structure has led recently to abandon the term "external urethral sphincter" because the urethral rhabdosphincter is not really external to the urethra, but more properly it surrounds the middle of the urethra. The term "urethral rhabdosphincter" has been therefore recommended.

In contrast to the levator ani muscles, the rhabdosphincter and perineal muscles embryologically develop from the cloaca, with a 2-week delay in striated muscular differentiation compared with the LA and other skeletal muscles [10].

We remember that they are completely separated from the LA by connective tissue [11].

Thus, the striated muscles associated with the viscera are quite distinct from the striated skeletal muscle of the pelvic floor.

1.3.2 Anal Sphincters

The prolongation of the circular muscle layer of the rectum, expanding caudally into the anal canal, becomes the internal anal sphincter (IAS), as reported by Varuna Raizada and Ravinder K. Mittal. In a parallel fashion, the longitudinal muscles of the rectum extend into the anal canal and end up as thin septa that penetrate into the puborectalis and external anal sphincter (EAS) muscles [12]. The autonomic nerves, sympathetic (spinal) nerves and parasympathetic (pelvic) nerves supply the IAS [13].

Sympathetic fibers originate from the lower thoracic ganglia and form the superior hypogastric plexus. Parasympathetic fibers originate from the 2nd, 3rd and 4th sacral nerves and form the inferior hypogastric plexus, which gives rise, from up to down to the superior middle and inferior rectal nerves: they innervate the rectum and the anal canal. These nerves synapse with the myenteric plexus of anal canal and the rectum. The majority of muscular tone of the IAS is myogenic, i.e., due to the properties of the smooth muscle itself. Angiotensin 2 and prostaglandin F2α play modulatory roles. Sympathetic nerves mediate IAS contraction through the stimulation of α and relaxation through β1, β2, and β3 adrenergic receptors.

Recent studies show that low affinity β3 receptors are predominant in the IAS. Anal sphincter relaxation is obtained by stimulation of parasympathetic pelvic nerves through nitric oxide containing neurons that are situated in the myenteric plexus. A more limited role is played by other potential inhibitory neurotransmitters like VIP (vasointestinal peptide) and by CO (carbon monoxide). Acetylcholine and substance P are the neuromediators for excitatory motoneurons located in the myenteric plexus of IAS.

The anatomy of external anal sphincter (EAS) has been largely investigated; it is formed by three parts: subcutaneous, superficial and deep ones. However, several investigators have found that the EAS is constituted only by the subcutaneous and superficial muscle bundles [14, 15].

The first is located caudal to the IAS, while the superficial one surrounds the distal part of the IAS. The deep portion is very thin and is often confused with the puborectalis muscle. 3D US and RMN studies have confirmed this anatomical point of view. EAS is attached to the perineal body and to the transverse perineal muscle anteriorly and to the anococcygeal region posteriorly. We must underline that the EAS is not completely circular in all its sections: the posterior part is indeed shorter in the inferior aspect. This should not be misconstrued as a muscle defect in the axial US and MR images of the lower anal canal.

The muscolaris propria of the rectum contains low threshold slowly adapting mechanoreceptors: they are involved in the detection of mechanical deformation of the myenteric ganglia and of the tension of the longitudinal rectal muscle. Mechanical deformations of the anal canal stimulate numerous free and organized nerve endings like Meissner, Krause and Golgi-Mazzoni corpuscles. They are exclusively sensitive and respond to light touch, pain and temperature. Afferent unmyelinated C and larger A fibers are responsible for neural transmission from the rectum and the anal canal to the spinal cord [16].

1.3.3 Urethra

Female urethra presents an outer layer that is formed by the striated muscular structure of the urogenital sphincter: it can be found in the middle three fifths of its length. In its upper two thirds, the sphincter-like fibers are disposed in a circular fashion. In the distal part, the fibers leave the urethra and surround the vaginal wall forming the urethrovaginal sphincter; other parts of the same muscle extend along the inferior pubic rami above the perineal membrane being indicated as the urethral compressor. This muscle is composed mainly by fibers of the slow-twitch type that are especially suited for maintaining a constant tone. When needed, a voluntary muscle activation of this striated muscle can increase the constrictive action on the urethra.

The urethral mucosa extends from the bladder (that presents a transitional epithelium) to the external meatus: its epithelium is primarily a nonkeratinizing squamous one. Among its characteristics we must underline that it is hormonally sensitive undergoing important changes with stimulation. This submucosal tissue is hormonally sensitive too and contains a rich vascular plexus. Groups of a specialized type of arteriovenous anastomoses have been found in it: they are thought to provide a watertight closure of the mucosa, also thanks to an increase in blood flow contemporary to an increase in abdominal vessel pressure. The considerable quantity of connective tissue that is interspersed within the muscle and submucosa contains collagen and elastin fibers: its function is that of a passive addiction to urethral closure. A series of glands, mostly predominant in the middle and lower third of the urethra, are found in the submucosal space, mainly along its vaginal surface. Therefore we can conclude that the admixture of the smooth and striated muscle, connective tissue, mucosa, and submucosa accounts for the urethral functional sphincter. This sphincter needs obviously an intact neural control to provide the watertight closure of the urethral lumen, the compression of the wall around the lumen, and to create a sophisticated means for compensating abdominal pressure changes.

1.3.4 Pelvic Floor Imaging

The anatomy and the functions of pelvic floor muscles has been recently deeply investigated with MRI and 3D US, so that novel insights have been reached and diffused. After that, muscles themselves have been analyzed during contraction and defecation with ultrafast CT scanning [17]. These studies demonstrated that the changes of pelvic floor hiatus are in relationship with puborectalis activity, being smaller during contraction and larger during defecation (Figs. 1.4 and 1.5). The changes in the pelvic floor hiatus size are predominantly related to the puborectalis muscle and they reflect the constrictor function of pelvic floor. On the contrary the other muscles, i.e., pubococcygeus, ischiococcygeus, and ileococcygeus muscles, are mainly responsible for pelvic floor and levator plate ascent and descent. The anorectal angle becomes acute and moves cephalad

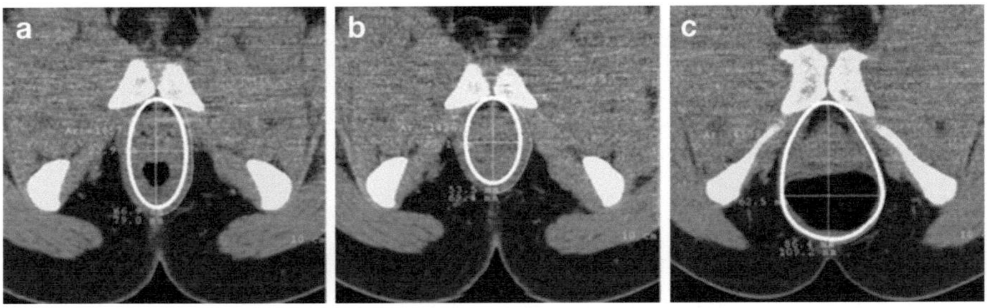

Fig. 1.4 Seated CT defecography, axial images of puborectalis at rest (**a**), squeeze (**b**), and defecation (**c**). Note that the pelvic floor hiatus becomes smaller during squeeze and larger during defecation (Adapted from Li D, Guo M. Morphology of the levator ani muscle. *Dis Colon Rectum*. Nov 2007;50(11):1831–1839, with permission)

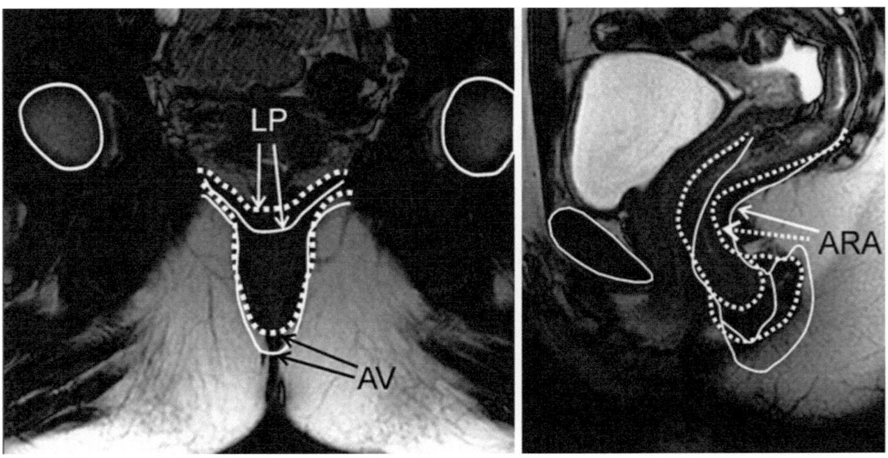

Fig. 1.5 Magnetic Resonance images (MRI) in the mid-sagittal and coronal planes: these images were obtained at rest (solid) and squeeze (dotted) and the images were overlapped to show the movements of various structures during squeeze. *LP* levator plate, *AV* anal verge, *ARA* ano-rectal angle

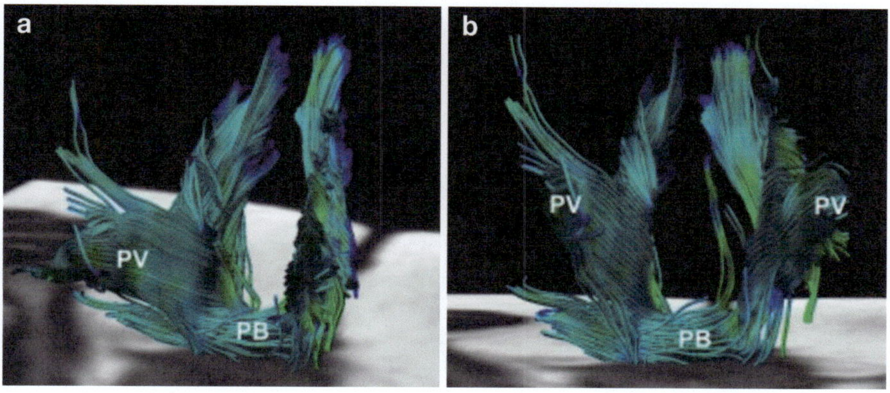

Fig. 1.6 Fiber tractography demonstrates the complex, multidirectional organization of the different pubovisceral (*PV*) muscle components in a 28-year-old female subject in both oblique-anterior (**a**) and anterior-posterior view (**b**). At the bottom of the pelvic floor transverse orientation of the fiber tracts are displayed matching the perineal body (*PB*) [18]

during pelvic floor contraction, while opposite changes occur during relaxation and defecation. Diffusion tension imaging (DTI) with fiber tractography has recently been used to analyze normal pelvic floor anatomy in a three-dimensional fashion (Fig. 1.6) [18].

1.4 Neuroanatomy

1.4.1 Puborectalis and Deep Pelvic Floor

Even if the concept that pelvic floor muscles are innervated from the S2, S3 and S4 sacral roots is commonly recognized, some controversies regard the innervation of levator ani muscle by the pudendal nerve. Varuna Raizada et al. reported that the middle layer of LA (puborectalis m.) is innervated by the pudendal nerve [19], whereas the deeper muscles (pubococcygeus, ileococcygeus and coccygeus) are innervated by the direct branches of sacral roots S3 and S4 [20]. Therefore they affirm that in human the levator ani muscle is innervated by the levator ani nerve [21]. It primarily arises from sacral spinal roots and travels along the intrapelvic face of the levator ani muscle with a high degree of variability in branching patterns. The consequence of this affirmation is that pudendal nerve damage may cause dysfunctions of puborectalis m, urethral and anal rhabdosphincters, responsible for urinary and fecal incontinence.

In humans, there is some controversy concerning whether or not the pudendal nerve also innervates the levator ani muscle [22, 23]. Several observations induce to describe a distinct special somatic motor innervation of the rhabdosphincters by the pudendal nerve vs. a typical skeletal motor innervation of the levator ani muscle by the levator ani nerve.

1.5 Peripheral Innervation of Urethral and Anal Rhabdosphincters

The motor neurons that innervate the striated muscle of the external urethral and the anal sphincters originate from a localized column of cells in the sacral spinal cord called Onuf's nucleus, expanding in humans from the second to third sacral segment (S2–S3) and occasionally into S1. Within Onuf's nucleus there is some spatial separation between motor neurons concerned with the control of the urethral and anal sphincters. Spinal motor neurons for the levator ani group of muscles seem to originate from S3–S5 segments and show some overlap [21]. Extensive studies of the urethral rhabdosphincter, anal rhabdosphincter, bulbocavernosus and ischiocavernosus muscles have shown that these muscles are innervated by the pudendal nerve. Traditionally the pudendal nerve is described as being derived from the S2–S4 anterior rami, but there may be some contribution from S1 and, possibly, little or no contribution from S4.

The nerve runs along the lateral aspect of the internal obturator and coccygeus muscles and through Alcock's canal (Fig. 1.7). In this portion, it branches into the inferior rectal nerve (for the anal rhabdosphincter), the perineal nerve (for the urethral rhabdosphincter, the bulbospongiosus muscle, the ischiocavernosus muscle, the superficial transverse perineal muscle and the labial skin), and the clitoris dorsal nerve. The branches of the perineal nerve are more superficial than the latter, and, in most cases, travel on the superior surface of the perineal musculature.

Therefore, Thor and de Groat [24] conclude that the pudendal nerve does not innervate to a significant degree the major muscles of the pelvic floor, i.e., iliococcygeus, pubococcygeus or coccygeus muscles. As regards morphology, levator ani motor neurons are similar to other skeletal motor neurons, showing large α and small γ neuronal cells distributed in the sacral ventral horn. One distinguishing feature, however, are some projections from levator ani motor neurons into Onuf's nucleus, the location of rhabdosphincter motor neurons: this ought to represent a mechanism of coordination between pelvic floor and rhabdosphincter functions. Unfortunately the position of the LA nerve at the level of the intrapelvic surface of the muscles may expose it to be damaged during the passage of fetal head during the 2nd stage of delivery, thus contributing to the correlations between parity and POP.

1.6 Reflex Activation of Urethral and Anal Rhabdosphincters

The activation of the segmental reflex by pelvic nerve stimulation related to bladder distension stimulates the urethral rhabdosphincter; therefore the afferent inputs from the urinary bladder have been emphasized as being of primary importance. This reflex is often referred to as the guarding reflex or continence reflex.

However, recent studies are placing greater emphasis on urethral afferent fibers [25], so that some researchers are speculating that the guarding reflex is actually activated more vigorously by urethral afferent fibers: if urine inadvertently begins to pass through the bladder neck and into the proximal urethra, a fast closure of the more distal urethral sphincter (against any urine loss) is requested more rapidly as compared with simple bladder distensions or increases in intravesical pressure. Since the pudendal nerve is composed even by some urethral afferent fibers (as well as rectal,

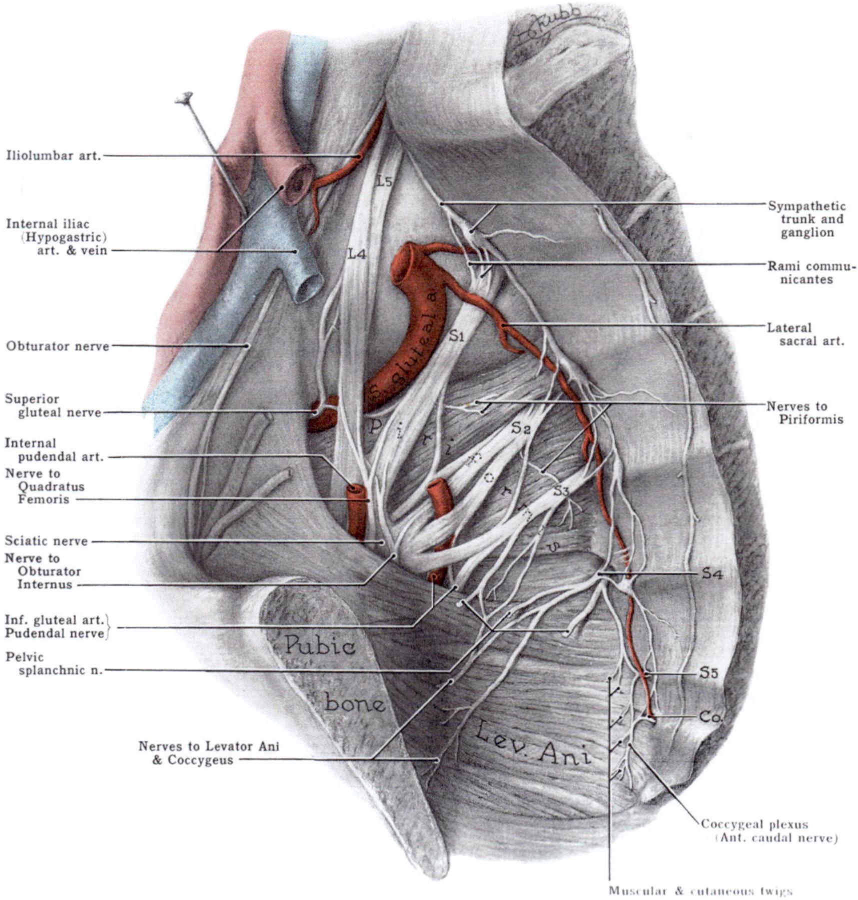

Fig. 1.7 Pelvic floor innervation (Grant (1962) An atlas of anatomy)

genital, and cutaneous ones), we may argue that the spinal urethral sphincter activation by pudendal afferent stimulation is also a manifestation of the guarding reflex.

Internal anal sphincter is innervated by autonomic sympathetic (spinal nerves) and parasympathetic (pelvic nerves) terminations. The former originate from the lower thoracic ganglia and form the superior hypogastric plexus, whereas the latter take origin from the 2nd, 3rd and 4th sacral roots to form the inferior hypogastric plexus, giving rise to the nerves that supply the rectum and the anal canal, that is the superior, middle and inferior rectal nerves.

1.7 Inhibition of Urethral Rhabdosphincter Reflexes During Voiding

Voluntary micturition is a behavior pattern that starts with the relaxation of the rhabdosphincter and the pelvic floor muscles. This can be detected as a disappearance of all EMG activity, which precedes detrusor contraction. The striated anal sphincter relaxes similarly with defecation and with micturition. Voluntary pelvic floor muscles contraction during voiding can lead to a stop of micturition, probably because of collateral connections to detrusor control nuclei. As a matter of fact descending inhibitory pathways for the detrusor have been often demonstrated. Bladder contractions are also inhibited by other reflexes that can be activated by afferent input from the pelvic floor muscles, perineal skin, and anorectum.

In addition to supraspinal inhibitory mechanisms, a spinal, urine storage reflex inhibitory center (SUSRIC) was found: it inhibits the somatic and the sympathetic urine storage reflexes, acting on the urethral rhabdosphincter and smooth muscle, respectively. Activation of SUSRIC by electrical stimulation of the pelvic nerve afferent fibers occurs simultaneously with the activation of the urethral rhabdosphincter reflex itself. Possibly the inhibition of rhabdosphincter activity by distension of the bladder represents a physiological corollary of the high-frequency electrical stimulation of pelvic nerve afferent fibers.

1.8 Levator Ani Innervation Damage in Childbirth and POP (see also Chap. 9)

It is well known that childbirth represents a risk factor for development of POP. Various studies have indicated that the damage to the innervation of the pelvic floor muscles may be the initial pathological cause for pelvic descent and prolapse [26–30]. Many other studies [31, 32] have underlined that levator ani nerve damage follows parturition in about 25 % of women with approximately one-third of those showing a persistent nerve damage at 6 months after parturition. On the contrary, women undergoing elective cesarean section (CS) (i.e., without preceding labor) showed no signs of levator ani nerve damage, while damage occurred in similar proportions of women who had CS after protracted labor as the ones with vaginal delivery, i.e., without CS. Furthermore, changes in function of the urethral rhabdosphincter were also associated with pregnancy itself (i.e., before labor), and these remained evident at 6 months after childbirth. Some experimental studies on squirrel monkeys indicate that, in nulliparous animals, the pelvic floor muscles play a minor role in providing visceral support, thus suggesting that the connective tissue plays the major role. On the other hand, after childbirth and consequent stretching of the pelvic connective tissue, the muscle may play a compensatory role. The levator ani muscle stretching might induce a reflex muscle activity and hypertrophy.

Other lesion mechanism than neurogenic and structural damage, such as muscle ischemia, may also be operative during childbirth. Although muscle weakness may be a common consequence of childbirth injury, it is the strength of muscle contraction that defines its functional integrity. Parous women with stress urinary incontinence (SUI) are subject to significant reduction of duration of motor unit recruitment, unilateral recruitment of reflex response in the pubococcygeal muscle and paradoxical inhibition of continuous firing of motor units in pelvic floor muscles activation on coughing.

Another mechanism through which the pelvic muscular support may facilitate pelvic organ prolapse is the avulsion of the puborectalis muscle from the pubic rami in the multipara. This kind of damage is present in 18–70 % of multiparous women, the majority of them showing POP on clinical examination [33–35].

Although not proven in studies, it is reasonable to assume that motor denervation is accompanied also by sensory denervation of the pelvic floor muscles. In addition to denervation injury there may be some further temporary “inhibitors” of pelvic floor muscles activity, such as periods of pain and discomfort after childbirth, increased by attempted pelvic floor muscles contraction.

All abovementioned factors may lead to a temporary disturbance of pelvic floor muscles neural control after childbirth. This, in combination with a particularly vulnerable pelvic floor neural control, might become persistent, even if the factors originally leading to the problem disappear.

1.8.1 Applied Physiology

Broadly, the pelvic floor muscles can be considered to have two important functions.

They provide (1) support and physiologic position to the pelvic viscera and (2) sphinteric or closure functions to urethra, vagina, and anal canal. In cadavers, the pelvic floor is shaped like a basin, but in living individuals its shape is like a dome [36, 37]. This changes of the pelvic floor during contraction, from a basin to dome shape, is due to the shortening of the three components of LA muscle. At the same time, conversion to the “dome” causes the lift of the pelvic viscera (including the rectum) in the cranial direction and provides mechanical support to all pelvic floor viscera. Therefore, the weakness of these muscles results in perineal descent. The puborectalis is generally considered to be fundamental in maintaining the anorectal angle [38]. Contraction of this muscle results in an acute anorectal angle; during defecation, its relaxation causes this angle to become obtuse. The anorectal angle can be analyzed with contrast defecography or MRI.

The puborectalis muscle is also involved in the anal canal closure mechanism, i.e., in anal canal pressure [39, 40].

In the proximal anal canal the closure pressures are related to the activity of IAS and puborectalis muscle, while, in the middle part, also to the contraction of the EAS, and, in the distal part, to that of the EAS alone.

The consequence of the contraction of the puborectalis muscle is the lifting up of the anal canal in the ventral or anterior direction causing the compression not only of the anal canal itself, but also of the vagina, and the urethra against the rear aspect of pubic symphysis. Therefore there would be a high-pressure zone in the vagina [41]. As a matter of fact the analysis of the vaginal high pressure zone reveals that the anterior and posterior pressures are higher than the lateral one, which suggests that vagina is compressed in the anterior-posterior direction by the contraction of puborectalis.

3D US images show that the dimensions of the pelvic floor hiatus become respectively smaller and larger with the contraction of the puborectalis [42]. During the pudendal nerve block, the pelvic floor hiatus is increased and the vaginal pressure is decreased.

1.9 Anorectal Function and Fecal Incontinence

Feces stored in the colon are transported past the rectosigmoid "physiological sphincter" into the normally empty rectum, which can store up to 300 ml of contents. Rectal distension causes regular contractions of the rectal wall, which is affected by the intrinsic nervous (myenteric) plexus, and prompts the desire to defecate. Stool entering the rectum is also detected by stretch receptors in the rectal wall and pelvic floor muscles; their discharge leads to the urge to defecate. It starts as an intermittent sensation, which becomes more and more constant. Contraction of the pelvic floor muscles may interrupt the process, probably by concomitant inhibitory influences to the defecatory neural "pattern generator," but also by mechanical insistence on sphincter contraction and the propelling of feces back to the sigmoid colon. The pelvic floor muscles are intimately involved in anorectal function. Apart from the "sensory" role of the pelvic floor muscles and the external anal sphincter function, the puborectalis muscle is thought to maintain the "anorectal angle," which facilitates continence, and has to be relaxed to allow defecation. Current concepts suggest that defecation requires increased rectal pressure coordinated with relaxation of the anal sphincters and pelvic floor muscles. Pelvic floor relaxation allows opening of the anorectal angle and perineal descent, facilitating fecal expulsion. Puborectalis and external anal sphincter activity during evacuation is generally inhibited. However, observations by EMG and defecography suggest that the puborectalis may not always relax during defecation in healthy subjects.

The etiology of fecal incontinence is nowadays considered multifactorial and can be divided into the following pathophysiologies (1) diarrhea or excessive amount of liquid stools, (2) rectal dysfunction, and (3) anal canal closure impairment. Three distinct anatomical structures such as IAS, EAS, and puborectalis muscle are involved in the physiological anal canal opening and closure. The interaction of these structures is fundamental in maintaining rectal continence under different circumstances and for different contents (solids, liquids, air). The specific role of each muscular component has been deeply investigated in several studies. They demonstrated that patients with fecal incontinence have often more than one defect in muscles responsible for continence, and that the severity of symptoms is related to the amount of defects in multiple muscles, confirming the credence to the "multi-hit hypothesis" of fecal incontinence.

1.10 Pelvic Floor Muscles and Constipation

The etiology of constipation, just like that of incontinence, is multifactorial. Two major types of constipation are commonly described: (1) slow transit type in which the movement of stools through the colon is reduced and (2) outlet obstruction type, in which there are some problems in emptying rectal contents. Outlet obstruction, related to pelvic floor dysfunction, accounts for 50 % or more cases of constipation in adults. Several names, i.e., anismus, pelvic floor dyssynergia, paradoxical puborectalis contraction, paradoxical sphincter contraction, and dyssynergic defecation have been commonly used to define this condition. Normally, during pushing for obtain defecation or in Valsalva maneuver, the respiratory diaphragm and the abdominal wall contract together, resulting in an increase in the intra-abdominal and rectal pressure.

Simultaneously, a relaxation of the pelvic floor and anal sphincter is observed. Analyzing the rectal and anal sphincter pressures, Rao classified dyssynergic defecation disorders into three different types.

Type 1 – increase in rectal pressure but anal sphincter contraction, Type 2 – no increase in the rectal pressure and in anal sphincter contraction, and Type 3 – increase in the rectal pressure but absent or incomplete sphincter relaxation.

Dyssynergic defecation is usually acquired in adult age, but in some cases symptoms begin in childhood: this fact suggests that the individual has never been able to learn correctly the defecation mechanism.

During defecation, pelvic floor muscles must undergo two modifications: (1) pelvic floor descent and (2) pelvic floor hiatus enlargement. The descent of pelvic floor muscles leads the anorectal angle below the pubococcygeal line (an imaginary line going from the lower end of pubic symphysis to the coccyx) and causes a widening of the pelvic floor hiatus with an increase in the anorectal angle. On the contrary, during pelvic floor contraction, the anorectal angle is pushed cranially and ventrally.

1.11 Mechanism of Urinary Continence

Urethral closure pressure must be greater than bladder pressure, both at rest and during increases in abdominal pressure to retain urine in the bladder. The resting tone of the urethral muscles maintains a favorable pressure relative to the bladder when urethral pressure exceeds the bladder pressure. During activities, a dynamic process increases urethral closure pressure to enhance urethral closure and maintain continence.

At rest continence is assured by a competent sphincter mechanism, including not only the striated and smooth muscle sphincter, but also the pelvic floor muscles and an adequate bladder storage function. Normal kinesiological sphincter EMG recordings show continuous activity of motor units at rest (as defined by continuous firing of motor unit potentials), which as a rule increase with increasing bladder fullness. Reflexes mediating excitatory outflow to the sphincters are organized at the spinal level (the guardian reflex).

The L region in the brainstem has also been called the "storage center". This area is thought to exert a continuous exiting effect on the Onuf's nucleus and thereby on the striated urinary sphincter during the storage phase; in humans it is probably part of a complex set of "nerve impulse pattern generators" for different coordinated motor activities such as breathing, coughing, straining, etc.

The dominant element in the urethral sphincter is the striated urogenital sphincter muscle, which contains a striated muscle in a circular configuration in the middle of the urethra and strap-like muscles distally. In its sphincteric portion, the urogenital sphincter muscle surrounds two orthogonally arranged smooth muscle layers and a vascular plexus that helps to maintain closure of the urethral lumen.

Anatomically the urethra can be divided longitudinally into percentiles, with the internal meatus representing point zero and the external meatus representing the 100th percentile. The urethra passes through the wall of the bladder at the level of the vesical neck where the detrusor muscle fibers extend below the internal urethra meatus to as far as the 15th percentile. The striated urethral sphincter muscle begins at the termination of the detrusor fibers and extends to the 64th percentile. It is circular in configuration and completely surrounds the smooth muscle of the urethral wall. Starting at the 54th percentile, the striated muscles of the urogenital diaphragm, the compressor urethrae and the urethrovaginal sphincter can be seen. They are continuous with the striated urethral sphincter and extend to the 76th percentile. Their fiber direction is no longer circular. The fibers of the compressor urethrae pass over the urethra to insert into the urogenital diaphragm near the pubic ramus. The urethrovaginal sphincter surrounds both the urethra and the vagina. The distal terminus of the urethra runs adjacent to, but does not connect with, the bulbocavernosus muscle. Functionally, the urethral muscles maintain continence in various ways. The U-shaped loop of the detrusor smooth muscle surrounds the proximal urethra, favoring its closure by constricting the lumen. The striated urethral sphincter is composed mainly of type 1 (slow twitch) fibers, which are well suited to maintaining constant tone as well as allowing voluntary increases in tone to provide additional continence protection. Distally, the recruitment of the striated muscle of the urethrovaginal sphincter and the compressor urethrae compress the lumen. The smooth muscle of the urethra may also play a role in determining stress continence. The lumen is surrounded by a prominent vascular plexus that is believed to contribute to continence by forming a watertight seal via coaptation of the mucosal surfaces. Surrounding this plexus is the inner longitudinal smooth muscle layer. This in turn is surrounded by a circular layer of striated muscle.

The attachments formed by the fascia connect the periurethral tissue and the anterior vaginal wall bilaterally to the arcus tendineus, whereas the muscular structures connect the periurethral tissue to the medial aspect of the levator ani [43]. Urethral support is warranted by a simultaneous action of fascia and muscles working together under the neural control. This musculofascial support forms a hammock against which the urethra is compressed during any increase in abdominal pressure.

The mechanism of continence is furthermore increased by the action of the urethral sphincter. Therefore the failure of one of the support components will not always be followed by a situation of stress incontinence, thanks to the compensatory effect of the other component. This may explain why urethral hypermobility does not produce incontinence in every woman. It may also explain why bulking agents, injected in the urethral wall, can be useful in women with urethral hypermobility, as they may improve urethral sphincter function.

During physical stress the urethral and anal sphincters may not be sufficient to passively withhold the pressures arising in the abdominal cavity, and hence within the bladder and lower rectum. Activation of the pelvic floor muscles is mandatory and may be perceived as occurring in two steps by two different activation processes. Coughing and sneezing are thought to be generated by individual pattern generators within the brainstem, and thus activation of pelvic floor muscles is a preset coactivation and not primarily a "reflex" reaction to increased intra-abdominal pressure. In addition there may be an additional reflex pelvic floor muscle response to increased abdominal pressure due to distension of muscles spindle within pelvic floor muscles.

The pelvic floor muscles can of course also be voluntarily activated anticipating an increase in abdominal pressure. Such timed voluntary activity may be learned.

Functionally, the levator ani muscle and the endopelvic fascia play an interactive role in maintaining continence. Impairments usually become evident when the system is stressed. The increase in abdominal pressure acts transversally across the urethra so that the anterior wall is deformed toward the posterior wall, and the lateral walls are deformed toward one another, thereby helping to close the urethral lumen and prevent leakage due to the concomitant increase in intravesical pressure. If there are breaks in the continuity of the endopelvic fascia or if the levator ani muscle is damaged, the supportive layer under the urethra will be more compliant and will require a smaller pressure increment to displace a given distance. During a cough, the levator ani muscle contracts simultaneously with the diaphragm and abdominal wall muscles to build abdominal pressure. This levator ani contraction helps to tense the suburethral fascial layer, thereby enhancing urethral compression. It also protects the connective tissue from undue stresses.

1.11.1 Urogenital Diaphragm (Perineal Membrane) and Perineal Body

The urogenital diaphragm is a strong, muscular membrane running between the symphysis pubis and ischial tuberosities across the triangular anterior part of the pelvic outlet. It lies external and inferior to the pelvic diaphragm. It contains three contiguous striated muscles: urethral compressor, urethral sphincter and urethrovaginalis sphincter; its inferior fascia is called the perineal membrane [44].

The perineal membrane is a complex three-dimensional structure composed by two distinct different regions, respectively dorsal and ventral; it is not indeed a simple trilaminar sheet perforated by pelvic viscera.

The more superficial ischiocavernosus and bulbocavernosus muscles, in conjunction with the thin layer of the superficial transverse perineal m. [45], complete the inferior aspect of the urogenital diaphragm. The structure fills the space between the inferior pubic rami and the perineal body, thus closing the urogenital (levator) hiatus; it supports and has a sphincter-like effect at the level of the distal vagina; moreover, thanks to its attachment to the periurethral striated muscles, it contributes to continence, providing also a structural support for the distal urethra. The posterior triangle around the anus does not present a corresponding diaphragm or a similar membrane.

The perineal body is a pyramidal fibromuscular structure with a cephalad apex situated in the midline between the anus and vagina, linked cranially to the rectovaginal septum. Below this, muscles and fascia converge and interlace medially. Attached to the perineal body are situated in the rectum, the vagina and the anal sphincter; it also contains smooth muscles, elastic fibers and nerve endings. During childbirth, the perineal body is heavily distended. Acquired weakness of the perineal body may predispose to defects such as rectocele and enterocele [46].

Using an MRI scan, three distinct perineal body regions are visible: (1) a superficial region situated at the level of the vestibular bulb, (2) a mid-region corresponding to the proximal end of the superficial transverse perineal muscle, and (3) a deeper region at the level of the mid-urethra and of the puborectalis muscle [47] (Fig. 1.8).

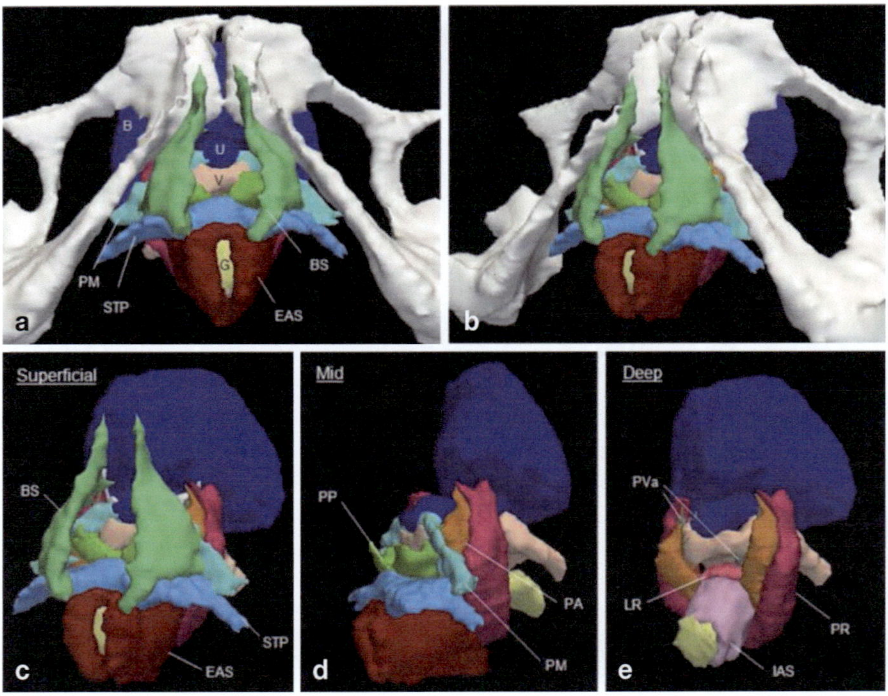

Fig. 1.8 (**a**) Dorsal lithotomy view and (**b**) left lateral aspect of same image. With removal of pelvic bones able to better appreciate superficial region (**c**) with BS, STP and EAS. (**d**) Lateral view with BS removed to illustrate mid region at proximal STP with PP, PM and PA. With removal of EAS, STP, PP, and PM can visualize deep region (**e**) with LR, PVa, PA. IAS visible with EAS removed. PVa muscle is barely visible lateral to the vagina in this image. PR-puborectalis, B-bladder, U-urethra, V-vagina, G-GI tract. © DeLancey 2010. Kindra A. Larson, et al. Am J Obstet Gynecol. ;203(5):494.e15-494.e21

1.12 Endopelvic Fascia and Connective Tissue Supports

This structure is situated just beneath the peritoneum and presents various thickenings in different areas. The endopelvic fascia, often called subserous fascia from an anatomical point of view, is continuous with the visceral one, which provides a sort of capsule containing pelvic organs and allows their displacements and possible changes in size. The distinct regions of this structure are indicated with different names, both ligaments and fascia. So we can distinguish, e.g., the pubourethral ligaments, the broad ligaments, the cardinal or Mackenrodt's ligaments, the uterosacral ligaments, and the arcus tendineus of the pelvic fascia.

1.12.1 Anterior Compartment Supports

The connective tissue supporting the urethra, bladder, and vagina takes origin from the arcus tendineus of the pelvic fascia [48, 49]. The pubourethral ligaments are situated anteriorly and consist of connective tissue structures that extend from the urethra to the pubic bone.

Because this represents an attachment of the lower third of the urethra to the pubis, it is postulated that exist two separate structures – one supporting the mid- or distal urethra and the other adjacent to the bladder neck – that must open it during voiding. The distal support is described as a connective tissue that links the vaginal wall and the periurethral tissue to the arcus tendineus of the pelvic fascia and to the levator ani muscles.

Urethropelvic ligaments running from the suburethral fascia at the level of bladder neck and proximal urethra to the levators and to arcus tendineus have been demonstrated using MRI imaging. DeLancey demonstrated the presence of a fascial layer situated suburethrally on the anterior vaginal wall. On the other hand, there is little actual endopelvic fascia at the level of the bladder base between the bladder and vaginal wall, so that the support is warranted by the lateral attachment of the vagina to the arcus tendineus of the pelvic fascia.

The pubocervical fascia has been described as a structure extending from the symphysis along the anterior vaginal wall to blend with the fascia surrounding the cervix. It is continuous with the pubococcygeus muscle laterally and it is suspended to the arcus tendineus too.

1.12.2 Apical Supports

The paracolpium and parametrium are the segments of connective tissues surrounding respectively the vagina and the uterus. In the mid-vagina, the paracolpium fuses laterally with the pelvic [28]. The cardinal ligaments (also called the ligaments of Mackenrodt) extend from the lateral aspects of the cervix and upper third of vagina to the lateral pelvic walls. They are connected to a large surface coming from the greater sciatic foramen over the piriformis muscles and from the region of the sacroiliac joint to the lateral side of sacrum. They represent a condensation of the lower parts of the broad ligaments. Laterally, they are also continuous with the connective tissue surrounding the hypogastric vessels. Medially, they are continuous with the paracolpium and parametrium and also with the connective tissue of the anterior vaginal wall, that is the pubocervical fascia.

Posterolaterally we found the uterosacral ligaments that are attached to the cervix and upper vaginal fornices. They attach to the presacral fascia in front of the sacroiliac joint. The connective tissue of the latter is continuous around the cervix with that of the cardinals. This complex of ligaments, i.e., cardinal and uterosacral ligaments, have the responsibility of keeping the uterus and upper vagina in their proper place over the levator plate.

1.12.3 Posterior Compartment Supports

The posterior vaginal wall, below the cardinals, is supported from both sides by the paracolpium, which is attached to the endopelvic fascia (referred to as rectovaginal fascia) and pelvic diaphragm. In this region there is only one attachment to the vagina, and there are not two distinct systems for the anterior and posterior vaginal sides. Therefore, when an increase of abdominal pressure pushes the vaginal downward, its attachments to the levator muscles prevent this downward movement.

Posteriorly, a rectovaginal septum, consisting of fibromuscular and elastic tissue and extending from the peritoneum to the perineal body has been described. We must remember that the peritoneal cavity extends to the cranial part of the perineal body during fetal life, but it is rapidly closed in early life. Its layers (known as the Denonvillier's fascia) probably become part of the rectovaginal septum that appears to be adherent to the surface of the posterior vaginal wall. This fascia forms the anterior margin of another potential space, the rectovaginal one. The rectovaginal septum, when intact, allows independent mobility of the rectum and the vagina. The mid-posterior vaginal wall is connected to the levator ani by the endopelvic fascia. These connections prevent the vagina from moving forward during the increases of abdominal pressure. The medial aspect of these parallel sheets is referred to as the rectal pillars.

In the distal vagina, 2–3 cm above the hymeneal ring, the vaginal wall is connected to surrounding structures without any intervening paracolpium. Anteriorly, the vagina is fused with the urethra and the connective tissue of the perineal structures of the urogenital diaphragm. It blends with the levator ani muscles laterally, while it fuses with the perineal body posteriorly. The rectovaginal fascia is thick [50] and therefore the vagina has no mobility in this area [51]. If the attachments of the perineal membrane to the perineal body is lacking as a consequence of fascial disruption, the bowel protrudes downward creating a posterior vaginal wall prolapse. The fascial supports for the rectum, that is the lateral rectal ligaments, extend from the posterolateral pelvic side wall (about at the level of the third sacral vertebra) to the rectum.

As outlined before, the cranial part of the vagina is suspended by the uterosacral ligaments. The compartment is rather wide at this point and there is not a direct contact between the genital tract and the pelvic walls.

In the mid-portion, the shape of the posterior compartment becomes smaller with the posterior vagina forming the ventral boundary, while the lateral margins are

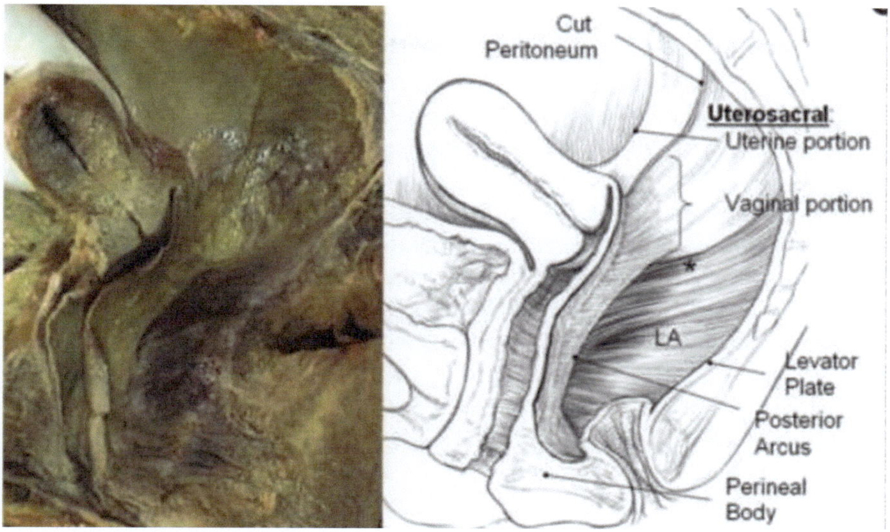

Fig. 1.9 Cadaver dissection (left) and illustration (right) of posterior compartment of a 56 year old multipararous female showing structural relationships after the rectum has been removed. Note the apical connections of the upper posterior vagina to the inside of the pelvic wall in a retroperitoneal position. These lie below the peritoneum and are dorsal and caudal to what is traditionally referred to as the uterosacral ligament. These structures are continuous with the posterior arcus tendineus fascia pelvis. At the distal end of the vagina the wall merges into the top of the perineal body. The lateral and dorsal margins of the compartment are formed by the levator ani muscles (LA) and the levator plate. The asterisk (*) denotes the region of the sacrospinous ligament overlain by the coccygeus muscle. © DeLancey 2007

formed by the pubococcygeus muscle and the dorsal aspect is formed by the puborectalis. The lateral margins of the vagina form a visible line indicated as the posterior arcus tendineus of pelvic fascia (Fig. 1.9).

Although the vagina in this portion is closer to the fibers of the levator ani, these structures are separated by a perivascular halo. In the lower portion of the posterior region, the perivascular halo is lost as the vagina appears fused to the adjacent levator ani, perineal body, and anus. The bottom of this compartment is marked where the subdivisions of the external anal sphincter and the perineal body can be seen [52].

1.13 Relationship Between the Pelvic Floor Muscles and the Fascial Support System

The interaction between the pelvic floor muscles and the supportive ligaments is critical to pelvic organ support. According to Ashton-Miller and DeLancey, as long as the levator ani muscles function to properly maintain closure of the genital hiatus, the ligaments and fascial structures supporting the pelvic organs are under minimal tension. The fasciae simply act to stabilize the organs in their position above the levator ani muscles. The constant tone maintained by the pelvic muscles relieves the tension placed on the endopelvic fascia. If the nerves to the levator ani muscles are damaged (such as during childbirth), the denervated muscles would atrophy and leave the responsibility of pelvic organ support to the endopelvic fascia alone. When the pelvic floor muscles relax or are damaged, the pelvic floor opens and the vagina lies between the zones of high abdominal pressure and low atmospheric pressure outside the body. In this situation it must be held in place by the suspensory ligaments. Although the ligaments can sustain these loads for short periods of time, if the pelvic floor muscles do not close the pelvic floor then the connective tissue will eventually fail and these ligaments gradually stretch under the constant load. This viscoelastic behavior leads to the development of pelvic organ prolapse. The attachment of the levator ani muscles into the perineal body is important and damage to this part of the levator ani muscle during delivery is one of the irreparable injuries to pelvic floor. It has been shown that up to 20 % of primiparous women have a visible defect in the levator ani muscle on MRI.

1.14 Summary and Conclusions

Pelvic floor muscles have two fundamental functions: they must provide (1) a physical support to the pelvic viscera and (2) the constrictor mechanism to the anal canal, vagina, and urethra. Newer imaging and physiological studies strongly suggest that these two functions are quite distinct and are likely related to different components of the pelvic floor muscles.

The pubococcygeus, iliococcygeus, and ischiococcygeus muscles are referred as providing the physical support or act as a "floor" for the pelvic viscera. On the other hand, the puborectalis muscle provides the closure mechanism for the anal canal, vagina, and urethra.

The urethra and anal canal have two separate sphincters of their own. As regards the anal canal these are the IAS and EAS, while for the urethra they are represented by the smooth sphincter situated at the bladder neck, and by the striated external urethral sphincter. Looking to the physiological studies, it appears that the puborectalis muscle may be considered as the 3rd constrictor, with a sphinteric function for the anal canal. The puborectalis serves also as a constrictor for the urethra itself. On the other hand, the vagina has only one closure mechanism, provided by the puborectalis portion or the pelvic floor muscle. We believe therefore that puborectalis muscle represents the real point of linkage among gastroenterologists, colorectal surgeons, urologists, and urogynecologists: all of them are the subspecialists taking care of patients with pelvic floor problems or dysfunctions. Recently this figure may be represented by a kind of new hyperspecialist named perineologist.

References

1. Strohbehn K (1998) Normal pelvic floor anatomy. Obstet Gynecol Clin North Am 25:683–705
2. Lawson JO (1974) Pelvic anatomy I: pelvic floor muscles. Ann R Coll Surg Engl 54:244–252
3. DeLancey JO, Delmas V (2004) Groos anatomy and functional anatomy of the pelvic floor. Elsevier Saunders, Philadelphia
4. Kearney R, Sawhney R, DeLancey JO (2004) Levator ani muscle anatomy evaluated by origin-insertion pairs. Obstet Gynecol 104:168–173

5. Salmons S et al (1995) Muscle. In: Williams PL, Bannister LH, Berry MM et al (eds) Gray's anatomy, 38th edn. Churchill Livingstone, New York, pp 737–900
6. DeLancey JO, Hurd WW (1998) Size of the urogenital hiatus in the levator ani muscles in normal women and women with pelvic organ prolapse. Obstet Gynecol 91:364–368
7. Dietz HP, Franco AV, Shek KL, Kirby A (2013) Avulsion injury and levator hiatal ballooning: two independent risk factors for prolapse? An observational study. Am J Obstet Gynecol 208(2):148.e1–148.e7. doi:10.1016/j.ajog.2012.12.006. Epub 2012 Dec 5
8. Fielding JR, Dumanli H, Schreyer AG et al (2000) MR-based three-dimensional modeling of the normal female pelvic floor in women: quantification of muscle mass. AJR Am J Roentgenol 174:657–660
9. Gilpin SA, Gosling JA, Smith AR, Warrell DW (1989) The pathogenesis of genitourinary prolapse and stress urinary incontinence of urine: a histological and histochemical study. Br J Obstet Gynaecol 96:15–23
10. Sebe P, Fritsch H, Oswald J, Schwentner C, Lunacek A, Bartsch G, Radmayr C (2005) Fetal development of the female external urinary sphincter complex: an anatomical and histological study. J Urol 173:1738–1742
11. Dorschner W, Biesold M, Schmidt F, Stolzenburg JU (1999) The dispute about the external sphincter and the urogenital diaphragm. J Urol 162:1942–1945
12. Raizada V, Mittal RK (2008) Pelvic floor anatomy and applied physiology. Gastroenterol Clin North Am 37(3):493–vii
13. Fritsch H, Brenner E, Lienemann A, Ludwikowski B (2002) Anal sphincter complex: reinterpreted morphology and its clinical relevance. Dis Colon Rectum 45(2):188–194 [PubMed]
14. Bogduk N (1996) Issues in anatomy: the external anal sphincter revisited. Aust N Z J Surg 66:626–629
15. Peschers UM, DeLancey JO, Fritsch H, Quint LE, Prince MR (1997) Cross-sectional imaging anatomy of the anal sphincters. Obstet Gynecol 90(5):839–844
16. Bharucha AE (2006) Pelvic floor: anatomy and function. Neurogastroenterol Motil 18(7):507–519
17. Li D, Guo M (2007) Morphology of the levator ani muscle. Dis Colon Rectum 50:1831–1839
18. Zijta FM, Froeling M, van der Paardt MP, Lakeman MME, Bipat S, Montauban van Swijndregt AD, Strijkers GJ, Nederveen AJ, Stoker J (2011) Feasibility of diffusion tensor imaging (DTI) with fibre tractography of the normal female pelvic floor. Eur Radiol 21(6):1243–1249
19. Guaderrama NM, Liu J, Nager CW et al (2005) Evidence for the innervation of pelvic floor muscles by the pudendal nerve. Obstet Gynecol 106:774–781
20. Dyck PJ, Thomas PK (2005) Autonomic and somatic systems to the anorectum and pelvic floor, 4th edn. Elsevier Saunders, Philadelphia
21. Barber MD, Bremer RE, Thor KB, Dolber PC, Kuehl TJ, Coates KW (2002) Innervation of the female levator ani muscles. Am J Obstet Gynecol 187:64–71
22. Grigorescu BA, Lazarou G, Olson TR, Downie SA, Powers K, Greston WM, Mikhail MS (2008) Innervation of the levator ani muscles: description of the nerve branches to the pubococcygeus, iliococcygeus, and puborectalis muscles. Int Urogynecol J Pelvic Floor Dysfunct 19:107–116
23. Wallner C, van Wissen J, Maas CP, Dabhoiwala NF, Deruiter MC, Lamers WH (2007) The contribution of the levator ani nerve and the pudendal nerve to the innervation of the levator ani muscles; a study in human fetuses. Eur Urol 54:1143–1144
24. Thor KB, de Groat WC (2010) Neural control of the female urethral and anal rhabdosphincters and pelvic floor muscles. Am J Physiol Regul Integr Comp Physiol 299(2):R416–R438
25. Hurtado EA, Smith PP, Smith CP, Boone TB, Somogyi GT (2008) Urethral afferent signaling leads to activation of the external urethral sphincter and abdominal wall muscles. Neurourol Urodyn 27:105
26. Allen RE, Hosker GL, Smith AR, Warrell DW (1990) Pelvic floor damage and childbirth: a neurophysiological study. Br J Obstet Gynaecol 97:770–779
27. Smith AR, Hosker GL, Warrell DW (1989) The role of partial denervation of the pelvic floor in the aetiology of genitourinary prolapse and stress incontinence of urine. A neurophysiological study. Br J Obstet Gynaecol 96:24–28
28. Snooks SJ, Swash M, Mathers SE, Henry MM (1990) Effect of vaginal delivery on the pelvic floor: a 5-year follow-up. Br J Surg 77:1358–1360

29. South MM, Stinnett SS, Sanders DB, Weidner AC (2009) Levator ani denervation and reinnervation 6 months after childbirth. Am J Obstet Gynecol 200:519.e1–519.e7
30. Weidner AC, Jamison MG, Branham V, South MM, Borawski KM, Romero AA (2006) Neuropathic injury to the levator ani occurs in 1 in 4 primiparous women. Am J Obstet Gynecol 195:1851–1856
31. Weidner AC, Sanders DB, Nandedkar SD, Bump RC (2000) Quantitative electromyographic analysis of levator ani and external anal sphincter muscles of nulliparous women. Am J Obstet Gynecol 183:1249–1256
32. Weidner AC, South MM, Sanders DB, Stinnett SS (2009) Change in urethral sphincter neuromuscular function during pregnancy persists after delivery. Am J Obstet Gynecol 201:529.e1–529.e6
33. Abdool Z, Shek KL, Dietz HP (2009) The effect of levator avulsion on hiatal dimension and function. Am J Obstet Gynecol 201(1):89.e1–89.e5
34. Dietz HP, Franco AV, Shek KL, Kirby A (2012) Avulsion injury and levator hiatal ballooning: two independent risk factors for prolapse? An observational study. Acta Obstet Gynecol Scand 91(2):211–214
35. Lammers K, Fütterer JJ, Inthout J, Prokop M, Vierhout ME, Kluivers KB (2013) Correlating signs and symptoms with pubovisceral muscle avulsions on magnetic resonance imaging. Am J Obstet Gynecol 208(2):148.e1–148.e7
36. Guo M, Li D (2007) Pelvic floor images: anatomy of the levator ani muscle. Dis Colon Rectum 50:1647–1655
37. Hjartardottir S, Nilsson J, Petersen C, Lingman G (1997) The female pelvic floor: a dome–not a basin. Acta Obstet Gynecol Scand 76:567–571
38. Bo K, Lilleas F, Talseth T, Hedland H (2001) Dynamic MRI of the pelvic floor muscles in an upright sitting position. Neurourol Urodyn 20:167–174
39. Jung SA, Pretorius DH, Weinstein M, Nager CW, Den-Boer D, Mittal RK (2008) Closure mechanism of the anal canal in women: assessed by three-dimensional ultrasound imaging. Dis Colon Rectum 51:932–939
40. Liu J, Guaderrama N, Nager CW, Pretorius DH, Master S, Mittal RK (2006) Functional correlates of anal canal anatomy: puborectalis muscle and anal canal pressure. Am J Gastroenterol 101:1092–1097
41. Guaderrama NM, Nager CW, Liu J, Pretorius DH, Mittal RK (2005) The vaginal pressure profile. Neurourol Urodyn 24:243–247
42. Weinstein MM, Jung SA, Pretorius DH, Nager CW, den Boer DJ, Mittal RK (2007) The reliability of puborectalis muscle measurements with 3-dimensional ultrasound imaging. Am J Obstet Gynecol 197(68):e61–e66
43. DeLancey JOL (1989) Pubovesical ligament: a separate structure from the urethral supports ('pubourethral ligaments'). Neurourol Urodyn 8:53–61
44. Stein TA, DeLancey JOL (2008) Structure of the perineal membrane in females: gross and microscopic anatomy. Obstet Gynecol 111(3):686–693
45. DeLancey JOL (1999) Structural anatomy of the posterior compartment as it relates to rectocele. Am J Obstet Gynecol 80:815–823
46. Nichols DH (1997) Central compartment defects. In: Rock JA, Thompson JD (eds) Te Linde's operative gynecology, 8th edn. Lippincott-Raven Publishers, Philadelphia, pp 1006–1030
47. Larson KA, Yousuf A, DeLancey JOL (2010) Perineal body anatomy in living women: 3-D analysis using thin-slice magnetic resonance imaging. Am J Obstet Gynecol 203(5):494.e15–494.e21
48. DeLancey JO (1994) Structural support of the urethra as it relates to stress urinary incontinence: the hammock hypothesis. Am J Obstet Gynecol 170:1713–1723
49. Weber AM, Walters MD (1997) Anterior vaginal prolapse: review of anatomy and techniques of surgical repair. Obstet Gynecol 89:311–318
50. Reiffenstuhl G (1993) Practical pelvic anatomy for the gynecologic surgeon. In: Nichols DH (ed) Gynecologic and obstetric surgery. Mosby, St. Louis, pp 26–71
51. DeLancey JOL (1992) Anatomic aspects of vaginal eversion after hysterectomy. Am J Obstet Gynecol 166:1717–1728
52. Yvonne HSU, Lewicky-Gaupp C, De Lancey JOL (2008) Posterior compartment anatomy as seen in MRI and 3-D reconstruction from asymptomatic nulliparas. Am J Obstet Gynecol 198(6):651.e1–651.e7

2 Perineal and Anal Sphincter Obstetric Injury

Gianfranco Minini

2.1 Introduction

Perineal trauma is a common event in first labour, affecting up 90 % of primigravidas and is sometimes associated with considerable postnatal morbidity and mortality [1].

The patients affected by perineal tears are at increased risk of recurrent severe perineal lacerations in subsequent deliveries [2].

Many of these patients develop subsequent anal incontinence and sexual dysfunctions despite adequate primary sphincter repair [3].

Around 3–4 % of women after childbirth suffer from faecal incontinence which is because of occult anal sphincter injury that has either been missed or it has been wrongly classified as a second-degree tear [4].

It is crucial to ensure that obstetric perineal injuries are recognized and repaired appropriately. Unfortunately, the majority of perineal and secondary anal sphincter repairs are the sequelae of unrecognized trauma or inadequate primary repair.

Missed diagnosis, lack of expertise, poor technique and inadequate training have all been suggested as reasons for the high rate of persistent symptoms after primary repair [5].

Identification of risk factors, vigilant monitoring and supervision by senior doctors during difficult/instrumental deliveries and good perineal support is recommended for minimizing the risk of perineal trauma as well as morbidity.

G. Minini
Department of Gynaecology, ICCB – Città di Brescia Clinic Institute, Brescia, Italy
e-mail: gianfrancominini@teletu.it

D. Riva, G. Minini (eds.), *Childbirth-Related Pelvic Floor Dysfunction: Risk Factors, Prevention, Evaluation, and Treatment*,
DOI 10.1007/978-3-319-18197-4_2

2.2 Classification of Perineal Lacerations

There is considerable inconsistency in the literature regarding the classification of perineal tears, especially relating to third- to fourth-degree tears.

In an attempt to standardize and produce the most descriptive classification, Sultan [6] originally proposed the classification of obstetric perineal and anal sphincter injuries (OASIS) shown in Table 2.1; this classification was later adopted by the Royal College of Obstetricians and Gynaecologists [7] and subsequently internationally accepted.

Rectal mucosal tear (buttonhole) without the involvement of the anal sphincter is rare and not included in this classification.

Based on this classification of perineal lacerations, the episiotomy is comparable to a second-degree tear.

A schematic representation of the anal sphincter is depicted in Fig. 2.1.

2.3 Epidemiology and Risk factors

The reported incidence of tears involving the anal sphincter occur in 1.7 % (2.9 % in primiparae) in centres where mediolateral episiotomy is practised, compared to 12–19 % (19 % in primiparae) in centres where midline episiotomy is practised [8].

Third- and fourth-degree lacerations can follow any type of vaginal delivery. Many studies have found that episiotomy is the factor with the strongest association with a third- or fourth-degree laceration [9]. Restrictive episiotomy policies appear to have a number of benefits compared to routine episiotomy policies. There is less posterior perineal trauma, suturing, and pain.

Certain other factors have been found to predispose to these lacerations (Table 2.2). A Cochrane Review of 10 trials [10] found that, compared to forceps, the vacuum extractor was associated with less maternal trauma, and therefore, less likely the associate with a third- or fourth-degree laceration. Factors not associated with these lacerations include body mass index (BMI), gestational age, marital status, pre-pregnant weight, weight gain in pregnancy, height, education, time of birth or physical fitness [11].

Table 2.1 Classification of perineal trauma

First degree: laceration of the vaginal epithelium or perineal skin only
Second degree: involvement of the vaginal epithelium, perineal skin and perineal muscles but not the anal sphincter
Third degree: disruption of the vaginal epithelium, perineal skin, perineal body and external anal sphincter (EAS) and/or internal anal sphincter (IAS):
3a: <50 % thickness of external sphincter torn
3b: >50 % thickness of external sphincter torn
3c: internal sphincter also torn
Fourth degree: a third-degree tear with disruption of the anal epithelium as well

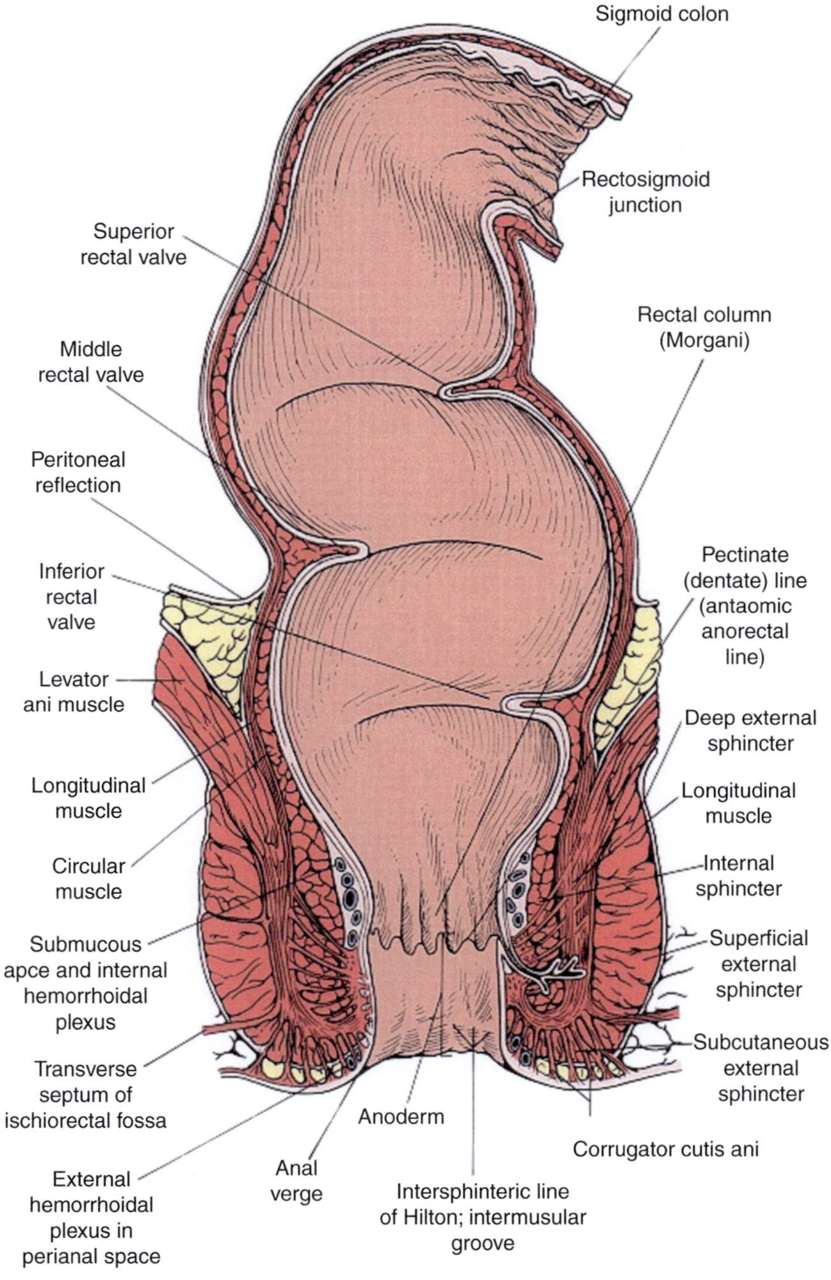

Fig. 2.1 Anatomy of the anus

Table 2.2 Risk factors associated with third- and fourth-degree lacerations

Anaesthesia (local and epidural)	Nulliparity
Asian or Pacific Islander ethnicity	Occiput transverse of occiput posterior position
Delivery with stirrups (delivery table, lithotomy)	Operative delivery (forceps > vacuum)
Routine episiotomy (midline > mediolateral)	Patient age (<21 years)
Increasing birth weight	Use of oxytocin
Increased second stage of labour	Birth weight >4 kg

Taking an overall risk of 1 % of vaginal deliveries, the reported factors are associated with this increased risk of a third-degree tear: birth weight over 4 kg, up to 2 %; persistent occipitoposterior position, up to 3 %; nulliparity, up to 4 %; induction of labour, up to 2 %; epidural analgesia, up to 2 %; second stage longer than 1 h, up to 4 %; shoulder dystocia, up to 4 %; midline episiotomy, up to 3 %; forceps delivery, up to 7 % [12].

A lower risk of third-degree tear is associated with a larger angle of episiotomy. In a prospective case-control study, there was a 50 % relative reduction in risk of sustaining third-degree tear observed for every 6° away from the perineal midline that an episiotomy was cut.

2.4 Clinical Aspects

Vaginal delivery has been directly implicated as a major aetiological factor in urinary/faecal incontinence, dyspareunia and uterovaginal prolapse. Although some symptomatic women may present early, the majority tend to present much later, particularly during the perimenopausal years. This delay may be related to embarrassment or to other aggravating factors associated with pelvic floor weakness, such as ageing, oestrogen deficiency and progression of pelvic neuropathy. It is, therefore, crucial to ensure that obstetric anal sphincter injuries are recognized and repaired appropriately. Unfortunately, the majority of secondary perineal and sphincter repairs are the sequelae of unrecognized trauma or inadequate primary repair.

The sphincteric tears are complicated by genital fistulas in 3 % of cases. Maternal injury, as a consequence of failure to recognize and repair anal sphincter tear, is one of the most common causes of complaint and litigation arising in labour ward practice.

The anal incontinence affects the mothers physically and psychologically, and they are too embarrassed to seek help. Only 1/3 of patients with faecal incontinence had ever discussed the problem with a physician.

Table 2.3 reports the symptoms prevalence in third- and fourth-degree tears.

Table 2.3 Anal sphincter tears symptoms

Flatus incontinence	30 %
Liquid stool incontinence	30 %
Solid stool incontinence	4 %
Faecal urgency	26 %
All symptoms	15–57 %

Table 2.4 Preventive strategies

Allow time for adequate perineal thinning
Avoid an operative delivery (forceps > vacuum)
Avoid episiotomy
Perineal massage during the weeks before delivery in nulliparous
Lateral birth position
Perineal warm packs during the second stage

2.5 Prevention

In Table 2.4 are reported the best strategies to prevent a third- or fourth-degree laceration.

In particular, if one must perform an operative delivery, the use of vacuum extractor, rather than the forceps for assisted delivery, appears to reduce maternal morbidity.

2.6 Recognition and Identification of Obstetric Anal Sphincter Injury

In the RCOG second edition (2007) of the guideline about the management of third- and fourth-degree perineal tears, these statements are reported:

- All women having a vaginal delivery with evidence of genital tract trauma should be examined systematically to assess the severity of damage prior to suturing.
- All women having an operative vaginal delivery or who have experienced perineal injury should be examined by an experienced practitioner trained in the recognition and management of perineal tears.

With increased awareness and training, there appears to be an increase in the detection of obstetric anal sphincter injuries. One observational study showed that increased vigilance about anal sphincter injury can double the detection rate [13]. In another study where endoanal ultrasound was used immediately following delivery, the detection rate of anal sphincter injury was not significantly increased compared to clinical examination alone [14]. As there are clear difficulties with availability, access to staff trained in endoanal ultrasound on the labour ward, image quality and patient acceptability, the use of endoanal ultrasound in detecting anal sphincter injury immediately after delivery should be viewed as a research tool at present.

2.7 Surgical Techniques for Repairing Perineal Tears

It is essential that the full extent of the laceration is discerned, including extension of the laceration and 'button holes' defecting into the rectal mucosa. A careful rectal examination should be performed with the use of index finger by elevating the anterior rectal wall into the vagina. It is often useful to place a pad (usually a long pack of gauze pad) high into the vagina to prevent blood from the uterus of obscuring the view. The internal anal sphincter (IAS) is paler in colour than the external anal sphincter (EAS) and normally its distal end lies a few mm proximal to the distal end of EAS, but under general or spinal anaesthesia the distal end of IAS may be at a lower level.

Where the Internal Anal Sphincter can be identified, it is advisable to be repaired separately with interrupted sutures. The size of suture must be such as 3-0 PDS and 2-0 Vicryl which may cause less irritation and discomfort.

Regarding repair of the external anal sphincter, there are two surgical techniques: the overlapping and the end-to-end (approximation) method. The ends of the sphincter must be clearly identified and grasped with Allis clamps.

The end-to-end technique is used to bring the ends of the sphincter together using interrupted sutures placed through the capsule and muscle [15].

Allis clamps are placed on each end of the External Anal Sphincter. Monofilament sutures such as polydiaxanone (PDS) or modern braided interrupted sutures such as polyglactin (Vicryl) are placed at 'posterior, inferior, superior and anterior' side of sphincter. Recent evidence suggests that end-to-end repairs have poorer anatomic and functional outcomes than was previously believed [16].

An alternative technique is overlapping repair of the External Anal Sphincter. It brings together the ends of the sphincter with mattress suture and results in a larger surface area of tissue contact between the two torn ends. Dissection of the External Anal Sphincter from the surrounding tissue with Metzenbaum scissors may be required to achieve adequate length for the overlapping of the muscles. The suture is passed from top to bottom through the superior and inferior flaps, then from bottom to top through the inferior and superior flaps. The proximal end of the superior flap overlies the distal portion of the inferior flap. Two more sutures are placed in the same manner. After all three sutures are placed, they are each tied snugly, but without strangulation. When tied, the knots are on the top of the overlapped sphincter ends. Care must be taken to incorporate the muscle capsule in the closure [17]. The overlap technique is favoured by colorectal surgeons for secondary repair. For primary repair, either technique can be used [18].

Experience of the surgeon, operating theatre and its equipment, asepsis, lighting, operating instruments, anaesthesia, material and type of suture as well as medications are related with the effectiveness of the repair. A delay up to 8–12 h in primary repair does not seem to be detrimental to the functional outcome of the procedure.

2.8 Complications

It has been difficult to quantify the rates of complication from third- and fourth-degree lacerations due to the lack of uniformity in the literature in describing complications. Several studies provided individual rates which when combined gives a rough estimate of 15 % for the complication rate of third- and fourth-degree laceration repairs. The most common complications are listed in Table 2.5.

The factors that lead to complications are numerous, but the most common is breakdown secondary to infection. Poor approximations due to inadequate surgical technique or postoperative hematoma can also result in severe complications.

Although rare, necrotizing fasciitis of the perineum has a high rate of morbidity and mortality. Often occurring in patients with insulin-dependent diabetes, cancer or an immunosuppressive disorder, necrotizing fasciitis is a severe infection due to multiple bacterial pathogens, particularly anaerobes. This infection should be managed aggressively with surgical debridement and broad-spectrum antibiotics.

2.9 Postoperative Management

The use of broad-spectrum antibiotics and of postoperative laxatives is recommended following obstetric anal sphincter repair to reduce the incidence of postoperative infections and wound dehiscence.

Local protocols should be implemented regarding the use of antibiotics, laxatives, examination and follow-up of women with obstetric anal sphincter repair.

All women should be offered physiotherapy and pelvic-floor exercises for 6–12 weeks after obstetric anal sphincter repair, and should be reviewed 6–12 weeks postpartum by a consultant obstetrician and gynaecologist.

If a woman is experiencing incontinence or pain at follow-up, referral to a specialist gynaecologist or colorectal surgeon for endoanal ultrasonography

Table 2.5 Complications of third- and fourth-degree laceration repair

Anal incontinence
Dehiscence
Dyspareunia
Hematoma
Infection (superficial cellulitis, necrotizing fasciitis)
Perineal abscess
Rectocutaneous fistula
Rectovaginal fistula

and anorectal manometry should be considered. A small number of women may require referral to a colorectal surgeon for consideration of secondary sphincter repair.

2.10 Future Deliveries and Preconceptional Counselling

All women who sustained an obstetric anal sphincter injury in a previous pregnancy should be counselled about the risk of developing anal incontinence or worsening symptoms with subsequent vaginal delivery and should be advised that there is no evidence to support the role of prophylactic episiotomy in subsequent pregnancies.

There were no systematic reviews or randomized controlled trials to suggest the best method of delivery following obstetric anal sphincter injury. The risk of a subsequent vaginal delivery ranges between 17 and 24 % of worsening faecal symptoms. This seemed to occur particularly if there had been transient incontinence.

All women who have suffered an obstetric anal sphincter injury should be counselled at the booking visit regarding the mode of delivery and this should be clearly documented in the notes. If the woman is symptomatic or shows abnormal anorectal manometric or endoanal ultrasonographic features, it may be advisable to offer an elective caesarean section.

Risk management and potential litigation are important issues in the group with previous OASIS who elect to have vaginal deliveries. Informed consent is paramount and it is crucial that all these women are carefully examined by digital rectal examination following subsequent delivery and that any repair be conducted according to protocol by experienced trained personnel.

References

1. Kean L (2010) Perineal trauma. In: Luesly DM, Baker PN (eds) Obstetrics and gynaecology: an evidence based text for MRCOG, 2nd edn. Hodder Arnold, London, pp 447–456
2. Peleg D, Kennedy CM, Merril D, Zlatnik FJ (1999) Risk of repetition of severe perineal laceration. Obstet Gynecol 93:1021–1024
3. Sultan AH, Kamm MA, Hudson CN, Thomas JM, Bartram CI (1994) Third degree obstetric and sphincter tears: risk factors and outcome of primary repair. BMJ 308:887–891
4. Sultan AH, Kamm MA, Hudson CN, Thomas JM, Bartram CL (1993) Anal-sphincter disruption during vaginal delivery. N Engl J Med 329:1905–1911
5. Fernando RJ, Sultan AH, Radley S, Jones PW, Johanson RB (2002) Management of obstetric anal sphincteric injury: a systematic review and national practice survey. BCM Healt Serv Res 2:9
6. Sultan AH (1999) Obstetric perineal injury and anal incontinence. Clin Risk 5:193–196
7. Royal College of Obstetricians and Gynaecologists (2001) Management of third and fourth degree perineal tears following vaginal delivery. Guideline n° 29. RCOG Press, London
8. Hueston WJ (1996) Factors associated with the use of episiotomy during vaginal delivery. Obstet Gynecl 87:1001–1005
9. Delancey JO (2002) Episiotomy. In: Gilstrep LC, Cunningham FG, Vandorsten JP (eds) Operative obstetrics, 2nd edn. Appleton and Lange, Connecticut, pp 63–89
10. O'Mahony F, Hofmeyr GJ, Menon V (2010) Choice of instruments for assisted vaginal delivery. Cochrane Database Syst Rev 11:CD005455

11. Combs CA, Robertson PA, Laros RK (1990) Risk factors for third- degree and fourth-degree perineal lacerations in forceps and vacuum deliveries. Am J Obstet Gynecol 163:100–104
12. Christiansen LM, Bovbjerg VE, Mc Davitt EC (2003) Risk Factrs for perineal injury during delivery. Am J Obstet Gynecol 189:255–260
13. Km G, Paterson-Brown S (2002) Can we improve on the diagnosis of third degree tears? Eur J Obstet Gynecol Reprod Biol 101:19–21
14. Andrews V, Sultan AH, Thakar R, Jones PW (2006) Occult and sphincter injuries myth or reality? BJOG 113:195–200
15. Kammerer-Doak DN, Wesol AB, Rogers RG, Dominguez CE, Dorin MH (1999) A prospective cohort study of women after primary repair of obstetric anal sphincter laceration. Am J Obstet Gynecol 181:1317–1322
16. Williams A, Adams EJ, Tincello DG, Alfirevic Z, Walkinshaw SA, Richmond DH (2006) How to repair an anal sphincter injury after vaginal delivery: results of a randomized controlled trial. An Inter J Obstet Gynaecol 113:201–207
17. Sultan AH, Monga AK, Kumar D, Stanton SL (1999) Primary repair of obstetric anal sphincter rupture using the overlap technique. Br J Obstet Gynaecol 106:318–323
18. Daniilidis A et al (2012) Third degree perineal laceration. A review analysis. Open J Obstet Gynaecol 2:301–310

A Computerized Model of Pelvic Floor Muscles Physiology During Delivery

3

Maurizio Serati and Giorgio Bogani

Vaginal delivery is complex phenomena involving the activation of several muscles. In a normal condition, the descending fetal head meets resistance from the uterine cervix, the bone pelvic structures and the pelvic floor muscles [1]. Activation and stretch of pelvic muscles may influence vaginal delivery-related outcomes and the occurrence of pelvic floor dysfunctions. In fact, vaginal delivery (in particular the second stage of labour) is considered one of the main factors predicting for the occurrence of pelvic organs prolapse, urinary incontinence and chronic pelvic pain [1–4]. Hence, there is growing interest on this issue.

However, the interaction between the fetal head and the pelvic canal is not fully understood. In fact, owing to the difficulties in addressing these features in vivo, data on this issue are far from being clear. Several attempts have been done in order to clarify the biomechanical features occurring during a vaginal delivery. In particular, computerized-based models seem to be effective to study the process of vaginal delivery and the activation of pelvic floor muscles, thus allowing to clarify possible causes that may lead to muscle damages and pelvic floor dysfunctions [3–10].

Computerized-based models are quantitative analyses based on the principles of biomechanical practice. In the 1950s, a mathematical simulation called "finite element" was introduced to study the effects of mechanical load. This is a numerical method for finding approximate solutions to boundary value problems for partial differential equations. Variational methods are applied in order to reduce an error function and produce a stable solution. Accumulating evidence suggested that this method could be safely applied to investigate the effects that the descending fetus has on pelvic floor. In fact, this methodological analysis allows to quantify the biomechanical (direct or indirect) activation of pelvic muscles in different situations [3].

M. Serati, MD (✉) • G. Bogani, MD
Department of Obstetrics & Gynecology, Insubria University, Varese, Italy
e-mail: mauserati@hotmail.com

D. Riva, G. Minini (eds.), *Childbirth-Related Pelvic Floor Dysfunction: Risk Factors, Prevention, Evaluation, and Treatment*,
DOI 10.1007/978-3-319-18197-4_3

Parente et al. evaluated the applicability of this aforementioned method on parturition. In this population, the role of intra-partum pelvic floor muscle activation is unclear. Although the strongest pelvic muscles may protect the pelvic floor from delivery-related damages, no data support this assumption. As a matter of fact, we can speculate that excessive pelvic muscles training may promote resistance between the fetus and the pelvic canal, thus prolonging labour [3]. The authors, using a three-dimensional computational finite element model, studied the effects of muscle activation on the resistance against the fetal head descensus [3].

In this investigation, Parente et al. observed that pelvic floor muscles activation is related to an increase in resistance, thus supporting the assumption that muscles training increases the time of labour. The authors simulated the movements of the fetus (in vertex position) during labour. These movements included engagement, descent, flexion, internal rotation and extension. They performed three simulations using different values of muscles' strengths (i.e. passive, 5, 10 and 15 % of muscles activation). They observed that the maximum values of forces for passive, 5, 10 and 15 % in muscles' activation was about 26.5 N, 29.5 N, 33.2 N and 37.7 N, respectively [3].

In another study on this issue, the same study group investigated the influence of fetal head flexion during vaginal delivery. Using the same mathematical simulation of the above reported study (three-dimensional computational finite element model), they observed that increase in fetal flexion is associated with lower resistance against the fetal descent. By this point of view, sub-occipito-bregmatic diameter (complete fetal head flexion) reduces opposite forces in comparison to occipito-frontal diameter (poor fetal head flexion) [5]. Figure 3.1 displays the finite element model for the four degrees of head flexion.

Similarly, Lien et al. developed a three-dimensional computer model to predict muscles stretch at the time of vaginal delivery [6]. The authors used a model constructed from serial magnetic resonance images from a health nulliparous woman. The model was used to quantify pelvic floor muscles (i.e. iliococcygeus, pubococcygeus and puborectalis muscles) stretch induced by delivery [6]. They observed a sigmoidal relationship between fetal head descent and muscle stretch. The largest tissue strain reached a stretch ratio (tissue length under stretch/original tissue length) of 3.26 in medial pubococcygeus muscle, the shortest, most medial and ventral levator ani muscle. Ileococcygeus, pubococcygeus, and puborectalis muscles reached maximal stretch ratios of about 2.7, 2.5 and 2.3, respectively. Therefore, the authors concluded that medial pubococcygeus muscle is at greatest risk for stretch-related injury [6].

In another paper, focusing on three-dimensional computer-based simulation, Lien et al. studied the increase in pudendal nerve stretch during delivery [4]. They observed that the strain in perineal nerve branches innervating the anal sphincter, posterior labia and urethral sphincter reached values of 33 %, 15 % and 13 %, respectively. Interestingly, 25 % in nerves' strain is the known threshold to cause permanent damages in peripheral nerves [4]. Figure 3.2 shows pudendal nerve stretch occurring during the second stage of labour.

All these studies, based on computer technology, have several important clinical implications. Further computer-based evaluations are necessary to improve knowledge on this still unclear issue.

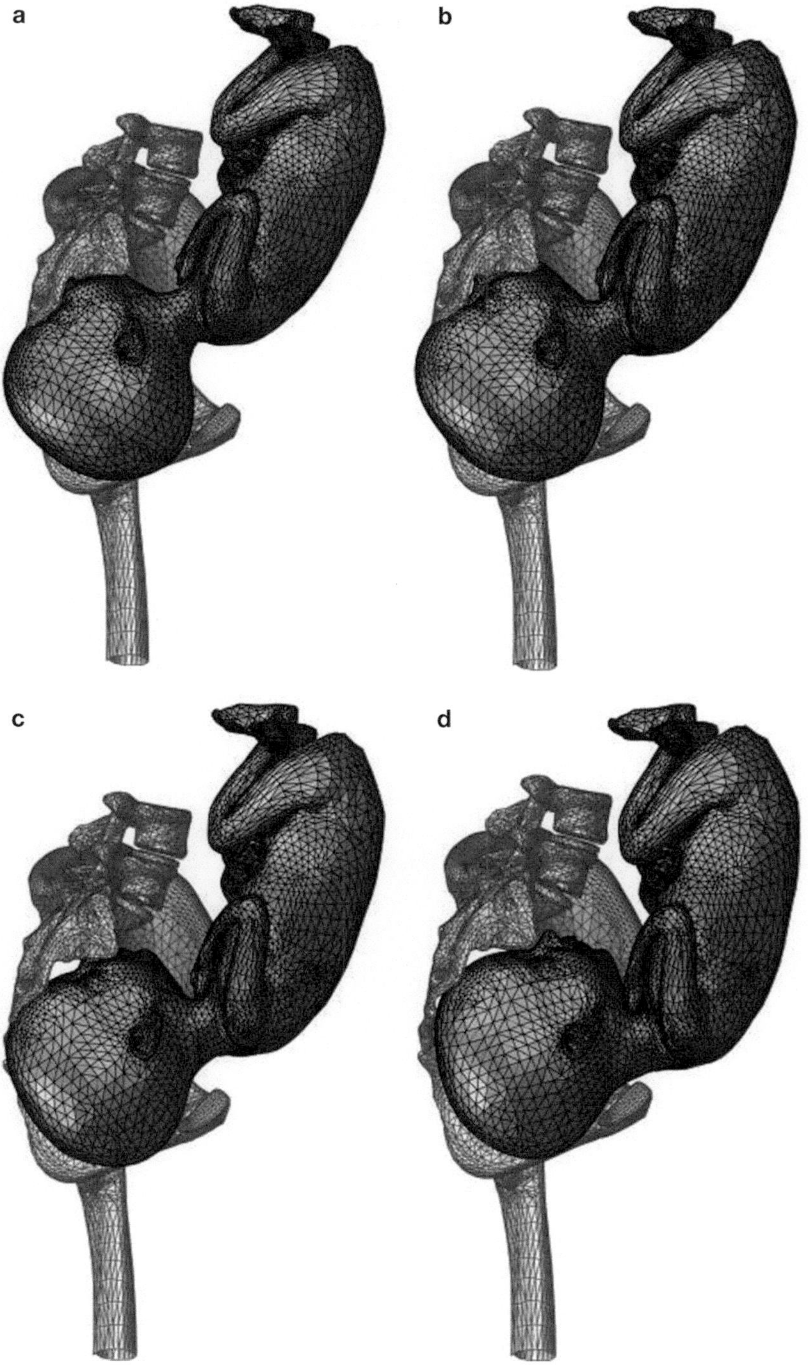

Fig. 3.1 Finite element with four degrees of head flexion. The fetal head flexion ranges from poor (**a**), moderate (**b**), advanced (**c**) and complete (**d**) flexion (From Parente et al. [5]. Used with permission)

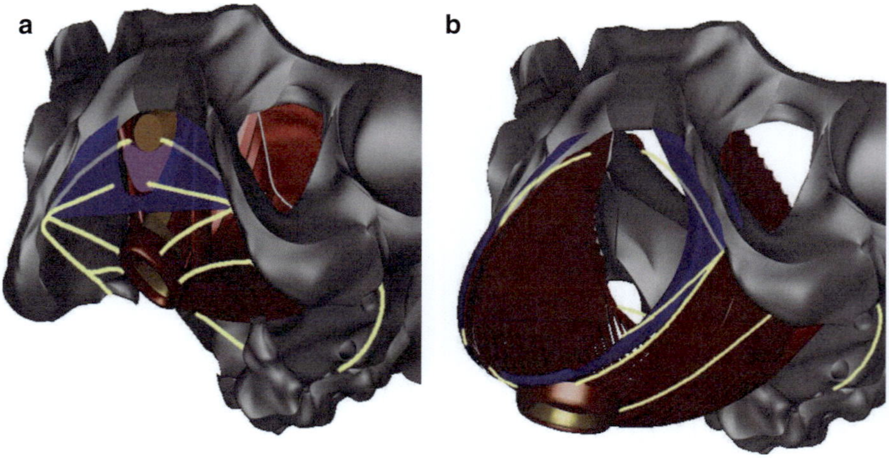

Fig. 3.2 Birth-related pudendal nerve stretch. The pudendal nerve (in *white*) and pelvic floor structure geometry at the beginning of the second stage of labour (**a**) and simulated pudendal nerve and pelvic floor muscle geometry at the end of the second stage of labour (**b**) are shown in an oblique lithotomy view (From Lien et al. [4]. Used with permission)

In conclusion, the embrace of computerized model allows to evaluate pelvic floor muscles physiology during delivery, thus improving knowledge of phenomena potentially affecting impaired intra and post delivery-related outcomes. Although there are inherent limitations of this methodology, consisting of non-in vivo evaluation of physiological pregnancy-related modification, these tools are effective to evaluate the effects of vaginal birth, thus improving intra- and post-partum outcomes. Further studies, involving more sophisticated software, are warranted in order to improve our knowledge on this issue.

References

1. Declercq E, Cunningham DK, Johnson C, Sakala C (2008) Mothers' reports of postpartum pain associated with vaginal and cesarean deliveries: results of a national survey. Birth 35: 16–24
2. Serati M, Bogani G, Sorice P, Braga A, Torella M, Salvatore S, Uccella S, Cromi A, Ghezzi F. Robot-assisted sacrocolpopexy for pelvic organ prolapse: a systematic review and meta-analysis of comparative studies. Eur Urol. 2014;66:303–18
3. Parente MP, Natal Jorge RM, Mascarenhas T, Silva-Filho AL (2010) The influence of pelvic muscle activation during vaginal delivery. Obstet Gynecol 115:804–808
4. Lien KC, Morgan DM, Delancey JO, Ashton-Miller JA (2005) Pudendal nerve stretch during vaginal birth: a 3D computer simulation. Am J Obstet Gynecol 192:1669–1676
5. Parente MP, Natal Jorge RM, Mascarenhas T, Fernandes AA, Silva-Filho AL (2010) Computational modeling approach to study the effects of fetal head flexion during vaginal delivery. Am J Obstet Gynecol 203:217.e1–217.e6
6. Lien KC, Mooney B, DeLancey JO, Ashton-Miller JA (2004) Levator ani muscle stretch induced by simulated vaginal birth. Obstet Gynecol 103:31–40

7. Parente MP, Natal Jorge RM, Mascarenhas T, Fernandes AA, Martins JA (2009) The influence of the material properties on the biomechanical behavior of the pelvic floor muscles during vaginal delivery. J Biomech 42:1301–1306
8. Li X, Kruger JA, Nash MP, Nielsen PM (2010) Effects of nonlinear muscle elasticity on pelvic floor mechanics during vaginal childbirth. J Biomech Eng 132:111010
9. Allen RH, Cha SL, Kranker LM, Johnson TL, Gurewitsch ED (2007) Comparing mechanical fetal response during descent, crowning, and restitution among deliveries with and without shoulder dystocia. Am J Obstet Gynecol 196:539.e1–539.e5
10. Hoyte L, Damaser MS, Warfield SK, Chukkapalli G, Majumdar A, Choi DJ, Trivedi A, Krysl P (2008) Quantity and distribution of levator ani stretch during simulated vaginal childbirth. Am J Obstet Gynecol 199:198.e1–198.e5

4 Clinical Approach to the Evaluation of Pelvic Floor Dysfunctions

Giancarlo Vignoli

Genitourinary changes following childbirth and pregnancy are common, and include urinary and anal incontinence, pelvic pain, sexual dysfunction and pelvic organ prolapse. At present, it is unclear whether or not these changes are a result of the pregnancy itself or the mode of delivery (caesarean section or vaginal birth). The exact mechanism of injury associating vaginal delivery with pelvic floor disorders is not known, but is likely multifactorial, potentially including mechanical and neurovascular injury to the pelvic floor [1, 2]. Operative vaginal delivery significantly increases the risk of PFDs. The evaluation and diagnosis of pelvic floor disorders, critical precursors of treatment, are feasible without specialized equipment. A specific history, voiding diary, focused physical exam and simple office tests provide sufficient data to diagnose most complaints. This approach frequently can be carried out without additional studies. In other cases, further investigations are needed to complete the work-up appropriately.

4.1 History

Traditionally, the goal of treatment is to restore normal pelvic anatomy. However, restoration of normal anatomy does not necessarily result in return to normal function of pelvic organs. This problem has led to a symptom-based approach for the evaluation and treatment of pelvic floor dysfunctions. During the office evaluation, it is, therefore, important to focus the history on patient's specific symptoms and to what degree these symptoms affect quality of life. An essential component of the

G. Vignoli
Functional Urology Unit, Casa Madre Fortunata Toniolo, Bologna,
Via Toscana 34, Bologna 40141, Italy
e-mail: vignoli.g@tiscali.it

D. Riva, G. Minini (eds.), *Childbirth-Related Pelvic Floor Dysfunction: Risk Factors, Prevention, Evaluation, and Treatment*,
DOI 10.1007/978-3-319-18197-4_4

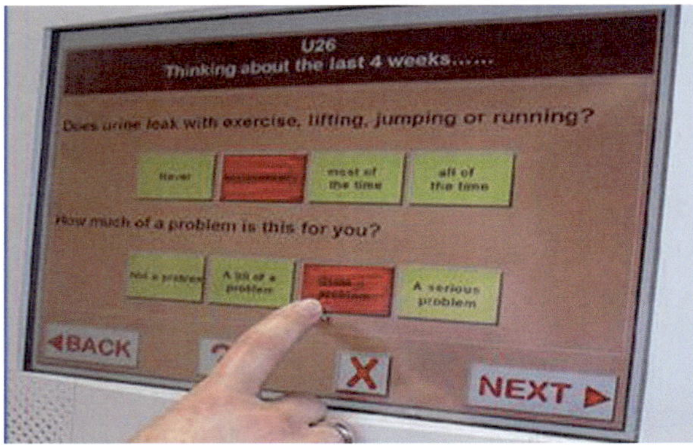

Fig. 4.1 e-PAQ-PF

pelvic floor history is a description of symptoms and quantification of their duration, frequency and severity, as well as any previous treatment the patient has undergone.

One way to facilitate a pelvic floor history is to give the patient a detailed questionnaire that can be completed prior to her initial office visit. The EPIQ is one of the first rigorously validate surveys developed to screen large population for the presence of PFDs [3]. This questionnaire generates scores for four pelvic floor disorders: stress urinary incontinence, overactive bladder, anal incontinence and pelvic organ prolapse.

In each case, a validated threshold is used to define women who meet criteria for the disorder. Scores greater than these threshold values have been shown to correspond to significant bother from pelvic floor.

To simplify collection data, an electronic form of questionnaire has been recently introduced [4]. e-PAQ-PF is an interactive electronic system that allows direct database entry via a touchscreen computer interface (Fig. 4.1). Both the original (14 domain) and enlarged (19 domain) version underwent psychometric testing in primary and secondary care, where it was found to be valid, reliable and acceptable.

The questionnaires are largely designed as outcome measures and are most useful in a research setting. The benefit to the practitioner not in a research environment is that a great deal of information about patient symptoms and the impact of those symptoms can be obtained in a short period of time.

4.1.1 Urinary Symptoms

Urinary symptoms range from frequency, urgency and nocturia, to dysuria and incontinence [5]. *Urge incontinence*, as its name implies, is typically preceded by an urge to void, and can involve a trigger such as opening home door, running water or cold temperature.

Stress incontinence generally occurs with sudden movements or increases in intra-abdominal pressure, such as those brought about by coughing, laughing, sneezing or running.

Table 4.1 The Questionnaire for female Urinary Incontinence Diagnosis (QUID) [6]

	None of the time	Rarely	Once in awhile	Often	Most of the time	All of the time
Do you leak urine (even small drops), wet yourself, or wet your pads or undergarments...						
1. When you *cough* or *sneeze*?	□	□	□	□	□	□
2. When you *bend down* or *lift something up*?	□	□	□	□	□	□
3. When you *walk quickly, jog* or *exercise*?	□	□	□	□	□	□
4. While you are *undressing* in order to use the *toilet*?	□	□	□	□	□	□
5. Do you get such a *strong and uncomfortable need* to urinate that you leak urine (even small drops) or wet yourself before reaching the toilet?	□	□	□	□	□	□
6. Do you have to *rush to the bathroom* because you get a *sudden, strong need* to urinate?	□	□	□	□	□	□

Scoring
Each item scores 0 (None of the time), 1 (Rarely), 2 (Once in awhile), 3 (Often), 4 (Most of the time) or 5 (All of the time). Responses to items 1, 2 and 3 are summed for the Stress score; and responses to items 4, 5 and 6 are summed for the Urge score

Many women with urinary incontinence have components of both stress and urge loss, otherwise called *mixed incontinence*. Few key questions may help in assessing the incontinence type (Table 4.1).

4.2 Implementation of Urinary Symptoms by Voiding Diary and Pad Test

Voiding diary is an inexpensive way to obtain information about a woman's daily bladder function. It is completed by the patient over a 24 h period and includes oral fluid intake, episodes of incontinence, associated activities and voids. Voiding volumes and times are recorded. The diary alone reveals that symptoms are attributable to excessive fluid intake, resulting in polyuria, or frequency due to OAB syndrome, and nocturia assignable to a nocturnal polyuria [7]. The severity of a patient's incontinence can be roughly assessed by the type and quantity of protection used (e.g. maxi pads or panty liners).

Pad test is a more objective method to determine the amount of urine loss [8]. The test may be short term or long term. Short-term test has the advantage of convenience and assured compliance. Long-term tests may be more representative of daily incontinence.

Short-term test generally involve the subject drinking a known volume of liquid or undergoing retrograde filling of the bladder. A preweighed sanitary pad is applied. The individual is instructed to perform specific activities such as coughing, running in place, bending and lifting, and handwashing. The testing interval can range from 15 min to 2 h. At the end of the test period, the pad is removed and weighed.

Long-term test is conducted under normal living conditions for 24–48 h. Each pad is preweighed and then weighed again after use by the patient at home, or alternatively, the pad is placed in an airtight plastic bag and weighed later by the clinicians.

According to ICS, the normal upper limits are 1 g for short-term test and 8 g for 24 h test.

The range for 'mild incontinence' is between 1.3 and 20 g, 'moderate incontinence' ranges from 21 to 74 g, and 'severe incontinence' is defined as 75 g or more in 24 h.

4.2.1 Pelvic Prolapse Symptoms

Minimal pelvic organ prolapse is usually asymptomatic. However, vaginal or uterine descent at or through the introitus can become symptomatic.

Symptoms of pelvic organ prolapse may include a sensation of vaginal fullness or pressure, sacral back pain with standing, vaginal spotting from ulceration of the protruding cervix or vagina, coital difficulty, lower abdominal discomfort and voiding and defecatory difficulties. Typically, the patient feels a bulge in the lower vagina or the cervix protruding through the vaginal introitus. Symptoms of voiding dysfunction, such as straining, hesitancy, intermittent flow, incomplete emptying, postvoid dribbling, are often associated to vaginal pressure or bulging.

4.2.2 Bowel Symptoms

Several faecal incontinence surveys attempt to quantify and qualify the severity of faecal incontinence. Two examples are the Fecal Incontinence Quality of Life Scale produced by Rockwood et al. and the Fecal Incontinence Questionnaire by Reilly et al. [9, 10]. Conversely, constipation surveys based on Rome III criteria seems less reliable [11].

However, patients who present for evaluation of bowel symptoms, particularly faecal incontinence, usually have had to overcome extreme embarrassment over their condition prior to their office visit. Care should be given to the manner in which the topic is approached in order to promote an open and comfortable discussion.

Questions about bowel function should include frequency of evacuations, faeces consistency, and presence of constipation. Faecal incontinence may include gas, liquid or solid stool.

Vaginal delivery is widely accepted as the most common predisposing factor to faecal incontinence in an otherwise young and healthy woman [7]. Vaginal delivery may result in internal or external anal sphincter disruption, or may cause more subtle damage to the pudendal nerve through overstretching and/or prolonged compression and ischaemia. An obstetric history should be taken carefully: prolonged second stage of labour, forceps delivery, significant tears and episiotomy, among other causes, are associated with increased risk for anal sphincter disruption and pudendal nerve injury.

Faecal urgency also must be differentiated from faecal incontinence because urgency may be related to medical problems other than anal sphincter disruption.

If constipation is the chief complaint, "splinting", i.e. the use of a finger pressing in the vagina or on the perineum during faecal evacuation, can be a sign of posterior prolapse or rectocele.

4.2.3 Sexual Symptoms

Sexual dysfunction includes disorders of sexual desire, arousal, orgasm and pain.

Like faecal incontinence, many patients are reluctant to proffer their sexual complaints, even when a sexual issue might be the very reason why the patient is seeking help. Thus, the responsibility of gathering a sexual history lies with the clinician, more than self-completion questionnaires. A good general strategy might be a step-by-step approach: first, by explaining the rationale for inquiring about sexual topics, while sympathizing with the patient reluctance to discuss intimate topics; then gradually introducing the topic of sexual issues, and finally addressing questions about the overall level of sexual interest and satisfaction and the presence of discomfort, pain or incontinence during sexual activity. Pain is the most common disorder in the post-partum as a consequence of perineal trauma. Although many women experience sexual problems in the post-partum period, the subject is still underexplored. Embarrassment and preoccupation with the newborn are some of the reasons why many women do not seek help.

4.3 Physical Examination

Once a complete history has been obtained, a focused physical examination should be performed. Attention should be centred on elements specific to pelvic floor disorders.

Inspection should consist of a careful visual examination of the perineal body and anus. The vagina should be checked with the aid of a speculum. Examination of the anal region may reveal skin tags, haemorrhoids, anal fissures, scars or chemical dermatitis. Rectal prolapse or fistulae may also be present.

After obstetric injuries, a discrete sphincter defect will almost always be anterior in location and be associated with loss of the perineal body or attenuation of the rectovaginal septum. Sometimes, however, the connective tissue of the perineal body is intact and only the sphincter has failed to heal. With an intact anal sphincter, the creases in the anal skin are arranged radially around the anal canal. When the

Fig 4.2 Points to measure during POP-Q pelvic examination

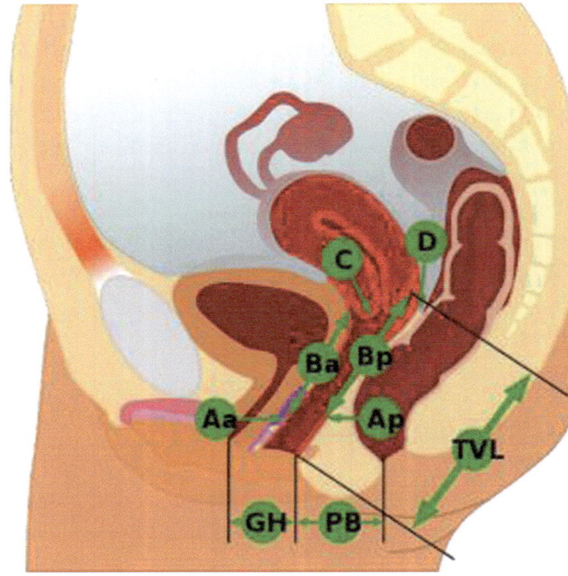

sphincter is disrupted and the perineal skin is intact, there is a classic dovetail appearance to the anus, in which the radial distribution of the anal skin creases is absent anteriorly.

4.3.1 Pelvic Prolapse Quantification (POPQ)

The POPQ system, introduced by the ICS in 1996, describes the location and severity of prolapse using segments of the vaginal wall and external genitalia, rather than the terms cystocele, rectocele and enterocele [12].

While the patient is straining, six specific sites are evaluated. Measure each site (in centimetres) in relation to the hymenal ring, which is a fixed, easily identified anatomic landmark. The hymenal ring is the zero point of reference. If a site is above the hymen, it is assigned a negative number; if it prolapses below the hymen, the measurement is positive.

The six POPQ sites are (Fig. 4.2) as follows:

- *Aa*: The point in the midline of the anterior vaginal wall 3 cm proximal to the urethral meatus, corresponding to the urethrovesical junction. By definition, the range of position Aa is −3 to +3.
- *Ba*: On the anterior vaginal wall, the most dependent position between point Aa and the vaginal cuff or anterior vaginal fornix.
- *C*: Cervix or vaginal cuff (posthysterectomy).
- *D*: Posterior fornix corresponding to the pouch of Douglas (this point is omitted in the absence of a cervix).

- *Ap*: The point in the midline of the posterior vaginal wall 3 cm proximal to the hymenal ring. By definition, the range of position Ap is −3 to +3.
- *Bp*: On the posterior vaginal wall, the most dependent position between Ap and the vaginal cuff or posterior fornix.

Two additional measurements are made in centimetres while the patient is straining:

- *GH*: The genital hiatus is measured from the midportion of the urethral meatus to the posterior margin of the genital hiatus.
- *PB*: The perineal body is measured between the posterior margin of the genital hiatus and the midportion of the anus.

While the patient is not straining, a ninth measurement is made:

- *TVL*: Total vaginal length is the greatest depth of the vagina.

Staging each compartment. When all nine of these measurements have been taken, a stage can be assigned to each compartment: anterior, apex (uterine or vault) and posterior. The stages are as follows:

- No prolapse is demonstrated. Points Aa, Ap, Ba and Bp are all at −3 cm and either point C or point D is within 2 cm of TVL. Stage 0
- The most distal portion of the prolapse is 1 cm above the level of the hymen (above −1). Stage I
- The most distal portion of the prolapse is 1 cm proximal to or distal to the hymen. Stage II
- The most distal portion of the prolapse is 1 cm below the hymen but protrudes no further than 2 cm less than the total vaginal length. Stage III.
- Complete eversion is present. Stage IV.

Unfortunately, the detail in making and recording nine measurements has been an impediment to more widespread clinical adoption of this system in favour of its 'rival', the Baden–Walker Halfway Scoring System. A POP–Q simplified system based on POP–Q with similar ordinal staging but with only four points measured instead of nine (Aa, Ba, C, D) has been developed. Evaluation of the interobserver reproducibility and intersystems reliability (in comparisons with the standard POP–Q system) showed good correlation [13]

4.4 Simple Office Tests

4.4.1 Postvoid Residual Urine (PVR)

The PVR should be measured within few minutes of voiding by catheterization or ultrasonography. When using ultrasound, transabdominal imaging is performed in the transverse and mid-sagittal planes. Once the measurements of the bladder's diameter in three planes (anterior-posterior, transverse and sagittal/longitudinal) are obtained, the volume can be calculated using the formula:

$$\text{Volume}(\text{mL}) = \text{height}(\text{cm}) \times \text{length}(\text{cm}) \times \text{width}(\text{cm}) \times 0.52$$

More recently, a dedicated ultrasound system has been developed for automatic measurement of PVR, thereby improving the accuracy over catheterization which has been largely abandoned in clinical practice.

In general, a PVR less than 50 ml is considered adequate bladder emptying and over 200 ml is considered inadequate emptying.

The documentation of the PVR is a prerequisite for any incontinence or anterior/apical prolapse procedure since the clinician will need this information to interpret any postoperative voiding difficulties and to counsel patients at increased risk of such difficulties.

4.4.2 Stress Test

A bladder stress test simulates the accidental release of urine (urinary incontinence) that may occur during cough, sneeze, laugh or exercise. Leakage of urine/water from the urethra coincident with coughing or straining after retrograde filling of the bladder with a known amount (usually 250–300 mL) of fluid demonstrates a positive stress test. This can be attempted first in the lithotomy position, but standing may be necessary to demonstrate leakage. A positive stress test performed with patient in supine position after emptying the bladder may indicate severe incontinence due to sphincteric damage. The demonstration of "stress incontinence" during simple bladder filling has a sensitivity of 88.1 % and a specificity of 77.1 % for the diagnosis of "genuine" stress incontinence, with a positive predictive value of 82 % and a negative predictive value of 84.4 % [14].

4.4.3 Q-Tip Test

In women with stress urinary incontinence, it is important to determine whether urethral hypermobility is present, since most of the surgical interventions for stress incontinence are designed to increase support to this area.

A standard sterile cotton swab lubricated with anaesthetic jelly is passed through the urethra just to the level of the bladder neck. The axis of the applicator is observed at rest and with coughing or Valsalva manoeuvre. A positive straining angle of 30° or greater from the horizontal indicates urethrovesical junction (UVJ) hypermobility. A straining angle of less than 30° indicates adequate UVJ support or hypomobility. The Q-tip test, however, is a quite inaccurate test. Compared with ultrasound measurements, it shows a sensitivity of 25 %, specificity of 78 %, positive predictive value of 67 %, and negative predictive value of 37 %. Furthermore, it exhibits a wide inter-observer variability [15].

4.4.4 Neurourologic Examination

Urinary incontinence, faecal incontinence, urinary retention and other pelvic floor disorders may be the presenting symptoms of neurologic disease. As such, all women with these symptoms should undergo, at minimum, a screening lumbosacral neurologic examination. This screening examination should include assessments of anal sphincter resting tone, voluntary anal contraction and perineal sensation. This simple screening examination can be performed quickly and easily as part of the gynaecologic examination. When abnormalities are noted, or when an individual is suspected of having neurologic dysfunction, a comprehensive neurologic examination with particular emphasis on the lumbosacral nerve roots should be performed.

4.4.5 Evaluation of Pelvic Floor Muscle Strength

The assessment of the strength of the pelvic-floor musculature is done by placing one or two fingers in the vagina and instructing the patient to contract the pelvic floor muscles (i.e. the levator ani muscles). The ability to contract these muscles as well as the strength, symmetry and duration of the contraction are assessed [16].

The strength of the contraction can be subjectively graded with a modified Oxford scale (0 = no contraction, 1 = flicker, 2 = weak, 3 = moderate, 4 = good, 5 = strong).

The evaluation of pelvic floor muscles is mandatory when a PFMT programme is planned.

4.5 Indications for Further Evaluation

The role of urodynamics in women with stress urinary incontinence remains controversial. Two recently published randomized controlled trials, the Value of Urodynamic Evaluation (ValUE) in the USA and the Value of Urodynamics prior to Stress Incontinence Surgery (VUSIS) in the Netherlands [17, 18], do not support the routine use of urodynamics before surgery in women likely to have genuine stress incontinence since it does not seem to improve significantly the outcome.

Detailed discussion on this hot topic is beyond the scope of this chapter. It is enough to say that urodynamics are merely tests that provide additional information regarding lower urinary tract symptoms. Although they would not be expected to improve the outcome of continence surgery, they offer valuable information to the surgeon and to the patient.

Stress urinary incontinence surgery may be performed without preoperative urodynamic studies in women with uncomplicated stress predominant urinary incontinence who have a positive office stress test, normal postvoid residual and normal urinalysis. However, in patients with more challenging issues, such as previous surgery for incontinence, concomitant prolapse, urge-predominant incontinence or neurologic disease urodynamics has still a pivotal role.

References

1. Handa VL, Blomquist JL, Knoepp LR, Hoskey KA, McDermott KC, Muñoz A (2011) Pelvic floor disorders 5–10 years after vaginal or cesarean childbirth. Obstet Gynecol 118:777–784
2. Memon H, Handa VL (2012) Pelvic floor disorders following vaginal or cesarean delivery. Curr Opin Obstet Gynecol 24:349–354
3. Lukacz ES, Lawrence JM, Buckwalter JG, Burchette RJ, Nager CW, Luber KM (2005) Epidemiology of prolapse and incontinence questionnaire: validation of a new epidemiologic survey. Int Urogynecol J Pelvic Floor Dysfunct 16:272–284
4. Jones GL, Radley SC, Lumb J, Farkas A (2009) Responsiveness of electronic personal assessment questionnaire – pelvic floor (e-PAQ-PF). Int Urogynecol J 20:557–564
5. Abrams P, Cardozo L, Fall M et al (2002) The standardisation of terminology of lower urinary tract function: report from the standardisation subcommittee of the International Continence Society. Neurourol Urodyn 21:167–178
6. Bradley CS, Rahn D, Nygaard IE et al (2010) The Questionnaire for Urinary Incontinence Diagnosis (QUID): validity and responsiveness to change in women undergoing non-surgical therapies for treatment of prevalent stress urinary incontinence. Neurourol Urodyn 29: 727–734
7. Kuo HC (2010) Interpreting voiding diary of patients with lower urinary tract symptoms. Incont Pelvic Floor Dysfunct 4:105–110
8. Rockwood TH, Church JM, Fleshman JW et al (2000) Fecal incontinence quality of life scale: quality of life instrument for patients with fecal incontinence. Dis Colon Rectum 43:9–16
9. Reilly WT, Talley NJ, Pemberton JH, Zinsmeister AR (2000) Validation of a questionnaire to assess fecal incontinence and associated risk factors: fecal incontinence questionnaire. Dis Colon Rectum 43:146–153
10. DiGesu GA, Panavi D, Kundi N et al (2010) Validity of the Rome III criteria in assessing constipation in women. Int Urogynecol J 21:1185–1193
11. Ryhammer AM, Djurhuus JC, Laurberg S (1999) Pad testing in incontinent women: a review. Int Uogynecol J Pelvic Floor Dysfunct 10:111–115
12. Bump RC, Mattiasson A, Bo K et al (1996) The standardization of terminology of female pelvic organ prolapse and pelvic floor dysfunction. Am J Obstet Gynecol 175:10–17
13. Swift S, Morris S (2006) Validation of a simplified technique for using the POP–Q pelvic organ prolapse classification system. Int Urogynecol J 17:615–620
14. Wall LL, Wiskind AK, Taylor PA (1994) Simple bladder filling with a cough stress test compared with subtracted cystometry for the diagnosis of urinary incontinence. Am J Obstet Gynecol 17:1472–1477
15. Caputo RM, Benson JT (1993) The Q-tip test and urethrovesical junction mobility. Obstet Gynecol 82:892–896
16. Bo K (2001) Vaginal palpation of pelvic floor muscle strength: inter-test reproducibility and comparison between palpation and vaginal squeeze pressure. Acta Obstet Gynecol Scand 80:883–887
17. Nager CW, Brubaker L, Litman HJ et al (2012) A randomized trial of urodynamic testing before stress-incontinence surgery. New Engl J Med 366:1987–1997
18. Van Leijsen SA, Kluivers KB, Mol BW et al (2012) Can preoperative urodynamic investigation be omitted in women with stress urinary incontinence? A non-inferiority randomized controlled trial. Neurourol Urodyn 31:1118–1123

Echographic Diagnosis of Childbirth-Related Pelvic Floor Injuries

5

Giulio A. Santoro and Maher A. Abbas

5.1 Introduction

During childbirth, pelvic organs (bladder, urethra, uterus, vagina, rectum, anal canal) and pelvic floor muscles, fascia, and ligaments may be damaged to some extent. Pelvic floor injuries can be identified immediately after childbirth or, more often, they may cause symptoms (urinary and fecal incontinence, voiding dysfunction, obstructed defecation, and pelvic organs prolapse) many years later. Damage to the anal sphincters is common but underdiagnosed at the time of delivery. Third- or fourth-degree tears are identified clinically after childbirth in 0.6–9 % of patients [1–6]. However, studies using two-dimensional endoanal ultrasonography (2D-EAUS) reported that trauma involving one or both sphincter muscles occurs in up to one-third of primiparous women [7], indeed, the true incidence of injury is probably closer to 11 %, as found using three-dimensional (3D) imaging modality [8–11]. In subsequent deliveries, it has been estimated that 8.5 % of women will develop sphincter laceration [12, 13]. Between one-third and two-thirds of women who sustain a recognized obstetric third-degree tear subsequently suffer from fecal incontinence (FI) [14]. In females who present with late onset FI, there is a high incidence of sphincter injury involving the external anal sphincter (EAS) in 90 % of cases and the internal anal sphincter (IAS) in 65 % of cases [14]. Injury to levator ani (LA) muscle as a result of vaginal birth has been documented using magnetic resonance imaging (MRI) [15–18], transperineal ultrasonography (TPUS) [19–25], and endovaginal ultrasonography (EVUS) [26–28]. It has been established that damage to this muscle, that represents an important element of the structural support mechanism in the pelvis, increases the risk of pelvic organ prolapse (POP) [29, 30].

G.A. Santoro, MD, PhD (✉) • M.A. Abbas, MD, FACS, FASCRS
Digestive Disease Institute, Cleveland Clinic Abu Dhabi,
Al-Maqam Tower, Sowwah Square, Al-Maryah Island, PO BOX 112412, Abu Dhabi, UAE
e-mail: Santorg@clevelandclinicabudhabi.ae; AbbasM@clevelandclinicabudhabi.ae

D. Riva, G. Minini (eds.), *Childbirth-Related Pelvic Floor Dysfunction: Risk Factors, Prevention, Evaluation, and Treatment*,
DOI 10.1007/978-3-319-18197-4_5

In this chapter, the different US techniques (2D/3D EAUS, EVUS, TPUS) to assess childbirth-related pelvic floor injuries and the clinical relevance of US diagnosis in the management of these conditions are described in detail [31].

5.2 Ultrasonographic Techniques

5.2.1 Transperineal Ultrasonography

Transperineal US is performed with the patient placed in the dorsal lithotomy, with the hips flexed and abducted, positioning a convex transducer translabial or on the perineum between the mons pubis and the anal margin (Fig. 5.1) [32]. Imaging is usually performed at rest, on maximal Valsalva maneuver, and on pelvic floor muscle contraction (PFMC). To avoid false negative results, transducer pressure on the perineum must be kept to a minimum consistent with good tissue contact, in order to allow full development of pelvic organ descent. Conventional convex transducers (main frequency between 3 and 6 MHz, field of view at least 70°) provide a 2D imaging of the pelvic floor. In the mid-sagittal plane, all anatomical structures (bladder, urethra, vaginal walls, anal canal, and rectum) between the posterior surface of the symphysis pubis (SP) and the posterior part of the LA are visualized [32]. Using volumetric probe (types: RAB 8-4, General Electric Kretz Ultrasound; AVV 531, Hitachi; V 8-4, Philips; 3D 4-7 EK, Medison), 3D and 4D TPUS imaging may be performed [21]. This transducer combines an electronic curved array of 4–8 MHz with mechanical sector technology, allowing fast motorized sweeps through the field of view. An

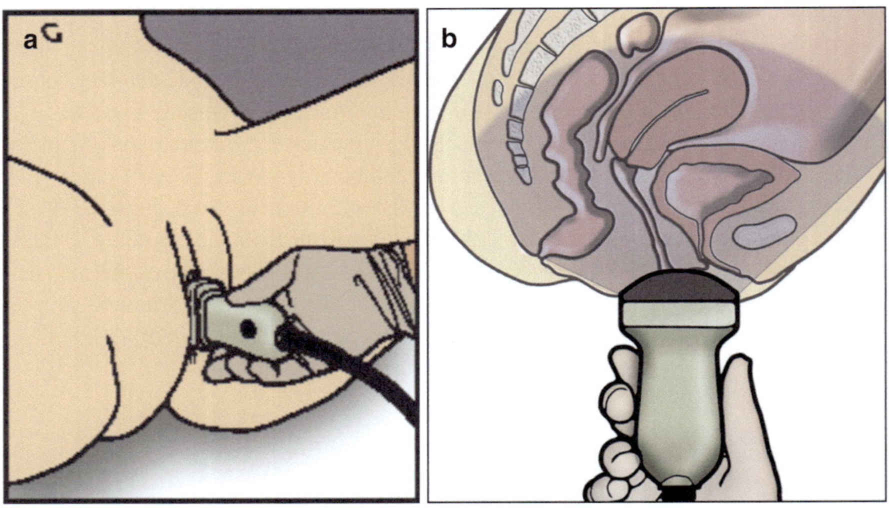

Fig. 5.1 Schematic illustrations of transperineal ultrasoud. (**a**) The patient is placed in the dorsal lithotomy, with the hips flexed and abducted, and the convex transducer is positioned translabial. (**b**) Field of view

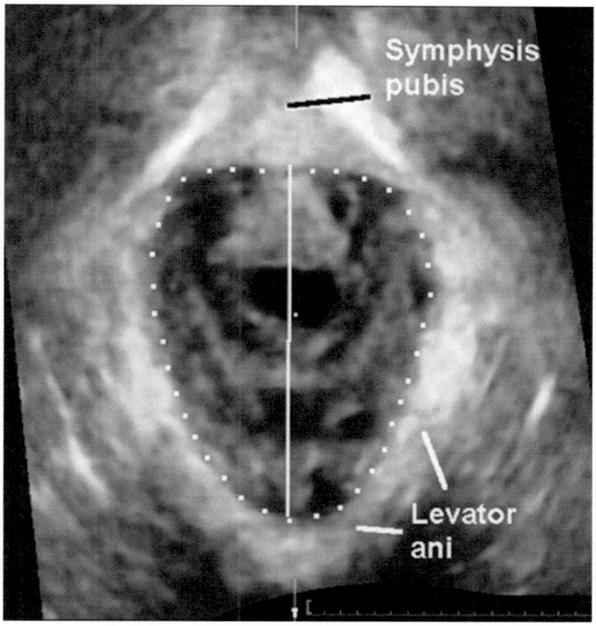

Fig. 5.2 3D transperineal ultrasound. In the reconstructed axial plane, the entire levator ani and its attachment to the inferior pubic rami are visualized. The diameter and area of the levator hiatus are measured in the plane of minimal anteroposterior dimension. (Courtesy of HP Dietz) and (from Santoro GA, Wieczorek AP, Bartram CI (eds) Pelvic floor disorders. Springer-Verlag Italia, Milan. With permission)

advantage of this technique, compared to 2D mode, is the opportunity to obtain tomographic or multislice imaging, e.g., in the reconstructed axial plane, in order to assess: (1) the entire puborectalis muscle (PR) and its attachment to the inferior pubic rami and to measure its dimensions in the plane of maximum muscle thickness; (2) the diameter and area of the levator hiatus (LH) in the plane of minimal anteroposterior dimension and the degree of hiatal distension on Valsalva (Fig. 5.2) [21, 33].

4D imaging indicates real-time acquisition of volume ultrasound data, which can then be visualized instantly in orthogonal planes or rendered volumes. Similar to DICOM viewer software used in radiology, offline analysis is possible on the actual system or on PC with the help of dedicated software [21, 33].

5.2.2 Endovaginal Ultrasonography

Endovaginal US may be performed with a high multifrequency (9–16 MHz), 360° rotational mechanical probe (type 2050, B-K Medical) or a radial electronic probe (type AR 54 AW, frequency: 5–10 MHz, Hitachi Medical Systems, Japan) [34]. The difference between these two transducers is the free-hand 3D acquisition with the electronic transducer, whereas the mechanical transducer has an internal automated motorized system that allows an acquisition of 300 aligned transaxial 2D images over a distance of 60 mm in 60 s, without any movement of the probe within the tissue. The set of 2D images is instantaneously reconstructed into a high-resolution 3D image for real-time manipulation and volume rendering. The 3D volume can

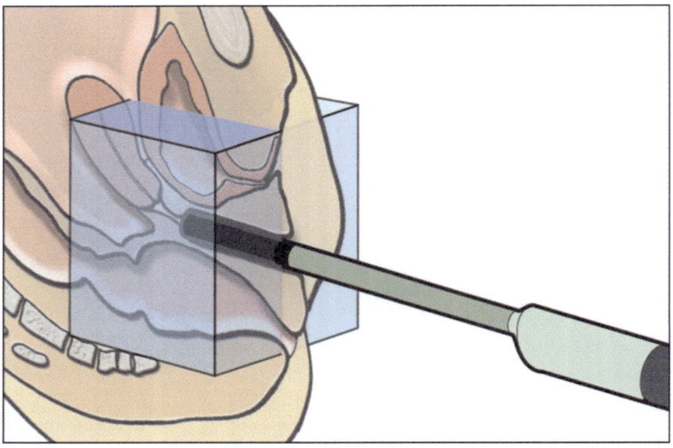

Fig. 5.3 Schematic illustrations of endovaginal ultrasound

also be archived for offline analysis on the ultrasonographic system or on PC with the help of a dedicated software [34].

During examination, the patient is placed in the dorsal lithotomy. It is important to keep the transducer inserted into the vagina in a neutral position, avoiding excessive pressure on surrounding structures that might distort the anatomy (Fig. 5.3). In the axial plane, 3D-EVUS provides a topographical overview of pelvic floor anatomy in four levels of assessment (Fig. 5.4) [34]:

- Level I: at the highest level, the bladder base can be seen anteriorly and the inferior third of the rectum posteriorly.
- Level II: corresponds to the bladder neck, the intramural region of the urethra, and the anorectal junction.
- Level III: corresponds to the midurethra and the upper third of the anal canal. At this level, the LA can be visualized as a multilayer hyperechoic sling coursing lateral to the vagina and posteriorly to the anal canal and attaching to the inferior pubic rami anteriorly (Fig. 5.5). The biometric indices of the LH can be measured in the axial plane of minimal hiatal dimensions: (1) anterior–posterior diameter: from the inferior border of the SP to the 6 o'clock inner margin of the LA; (2) latero-lateral diameter: taken on the widest part, perpendicular to LH anterior–posterior diameter; (3) LH area: calculated as the area within the LA inner perimeter enclosed by the inferior pubic rami and the inferior edge of the SP (Fig. 5.5) [35].
- Level IV: at the lowest level, the superficial perineal muscles (bulbospongiosus, ischiocavernosus, and superficial transverse perineal muscles), the perineal body (PB), the distal urethra, and the middle and inferior third of the anal canal can be visualized [36].

5.2.3 Endoanal Ultrasonography

Endoanal US is performed with high multifrequency, 360° rotational mechanical probe or radial electronic probe, already described for EVUS. During examination, the patient may be placed in the dorsal lithotomy, in the left lateral or in the prone

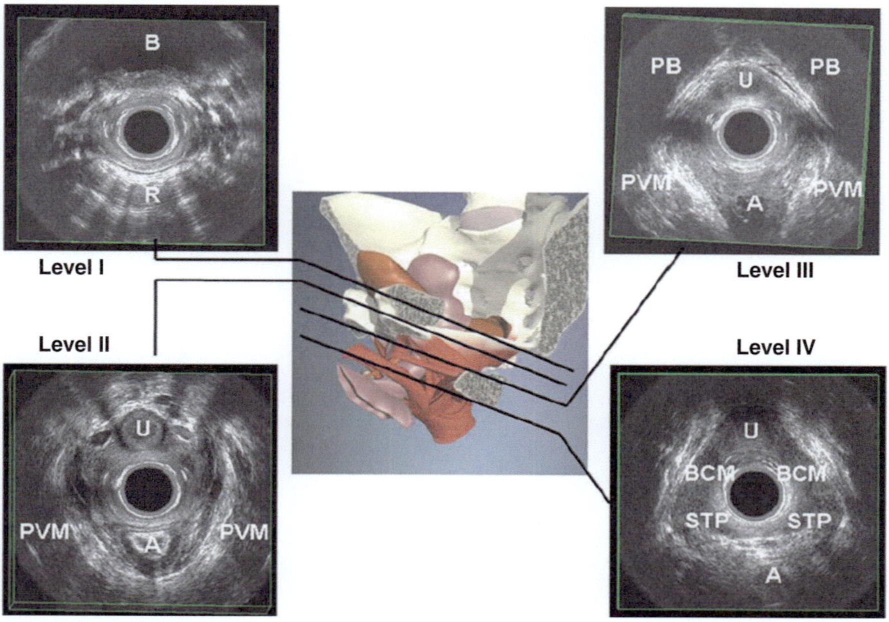

Fig. 5.4 Four levels of assessment of pelvic floor anatomy by using 3D endovaginal ultrasound (see text)

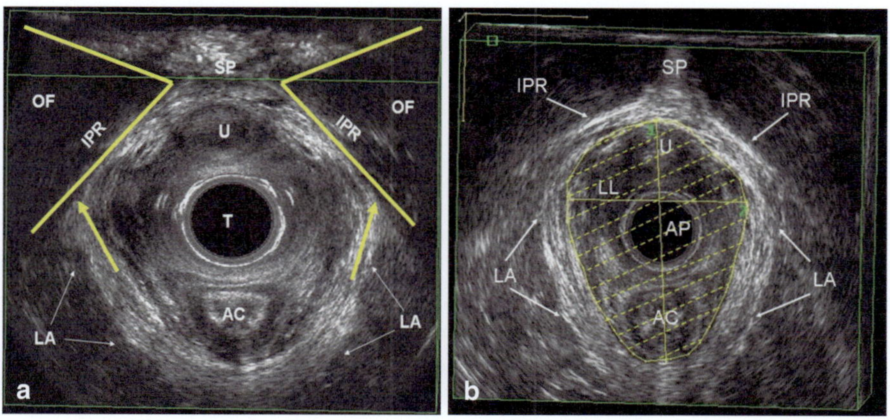

Fig. 5.5 3D endovaginal ultrasound. (**a**) Levator ani (*LA*) is visualized as a multilayer hyperechoic sling coursing lateral to the vagina and posteriorly to the anal canal (*AC*) and attaching to the inferior pubic rami (*IPR*) anteriorly. (**b**) The biometric indices of the levator hiatus are measured in the axial plane of minimal hiatal dimensions. *AP* Anterior–posterior diameter, *LL* latero-lateral diameter, *OF* obturator foramen, *SP* symphysis pubis, *T* transducer, *U* urethra

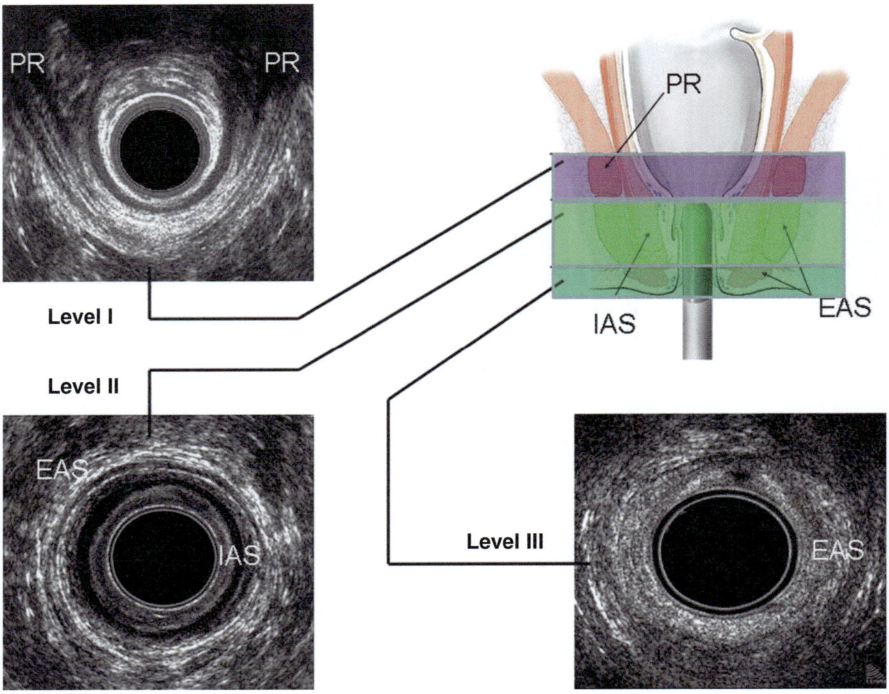

Fig. 5.6 Three levels of assessment of the anal canal by using 3D endoanal ultrasound (see text)

position. However, irrespective of the position, the transducer should be rotated so that the anterior aspect of the anal canal is superior on the screen. The length of recorded data should extend from the upper aspect of the PR to the anal verge. In the axial plane, three levels of assessment have been described (Fig. 5.6) [37]:

- Upper level: corresponds to the hyperechoic sling of the PR muscle and the concentric hypoechoic ring of the IAS. In males, the deep part of the EAS is also identified at this level,
- Middle level: the complete ring of the superficial EAS (concentric band of mixed echogenicity), the conjoined longitudinal layer, the complete ring of IAS, and the transverse perinei muscles are visualized.
- Lower level: corresponds to the subcutaneous part of the EAS.

3D-EAUS is useful in assessing the anatomic characteristics of the anal canal [38, 39]. The muscles of the lower and the upper part of the anal canal are different. At its upper end, the PR anchors the sphincter complex to the pubic rami. Anteriorly, the circular fibers of the deep part of the EAS are not recognizable in females, whereas in males the EAS is symmetrical at all levels of the anal canal. The IAS is not completely symmetric, either in thickness or termination. It can be traced superiorly into the circular muscle of the rectum, extending from the anorectal junction to approximately 1 cm below the dentate line. In the intersphincteric space, the smooth longitudinal muscle conjoins with striated muscle fibers from the LA, particularly the puboanalis, and a large fibroelastic element derived from the endopelvic fascia to form the conjoined longitudinal layer.

5.3 Echographic Diagnosis of Pelvic Floor Injuries

5.3.1 Anal Sphincter Damages

Obstetric injuries of the sphincter complex can be visualized in detail with EAUS [7–11]. All childbirth trauma affects the sphincters anterior to a horizontal line through the mid-canal. Any tear of the anal sphincters posterior to this line is due to some other etiology. Tears are defined by an interruption of the fibrillar echo texture. Scarring is characterized by loss of normal architecture, with an area of amorphous texture that usually has low reflectiveness. The number, circumferential (radial angle in degrees or in hours of the clock site) and longitudinal (proximal, distal, or full length) extension of the defect, presence of scarring, differences in echogenicity and thickness of the sphincters, and other local alteration should be carefully assessed and should always be described. The operator should identify if there is an isolated or combined lesions of the IAS and EAS according to OASIS classification [40, 41]: 1° degree = vaginal epithelium lesion; 2° degree = perineal muscles damage; 3° degree = anal sphincters involvement: 3a = <50 % EAS thickness; 3b => 50 % EAS thickness; 3c = IAS torn; 4° degree = 3° + anal epithelium torn. Defects of the IAS are easily recognized given the prominent appearance of the IAS in the mid-anal canal, and they appear as hyperechoic breaks in the normally hypoechoic ring. External sphincter tears from obstetric trauma always involve the upper sphincter, and may extend down throughout the length of the sphincter. The appearance of a defect is a break in the circumferential integrity of the mixed hyperechoic band of the EAS. A defect can have either a hypoechoic or hyperechoic density pattern. This corresponds to replacement of the normal striated muscle with granulation tissue, and fibrosis. The majority of obstetric injuries are associated with a single, large defect in the EAS anterior to the anal canal that can be linked to an additional division of the IAS (Fig. 5.7).

EAUS has an important role in detecting clinically "occult" anal sphincter injuries after a vaginal delivery. In a meta-analysis of 717 vaginal deliveries, Oberwalder et al. [42] found an incidence of occult sphincter damage of 26.9 % among a sample of 462 primiparous women and a rate of 8.5 % new defects in the group of 255 multiparas. In one-third of these (29.7 %), postpartum sphincter damage was symptomatic. As shown in this meta-analysis, the probability that postpartum FI will be associated with anal sphincter defect is 77–83 %. This analysis included five studies where EAUS was the only imaging technique used. In another study, Oberwalder et al. [14] reported that FI related to sphincter lesions is likely to occur even in an elderly population of women who experienced vaginal deliveries earlier in life. They found that 71 % of women with late onset FI (median age 61.5 years) had

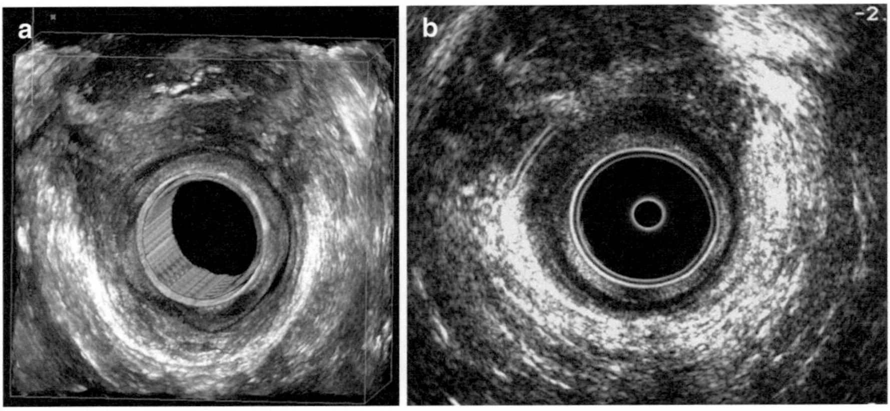

Fig. 5.7 Endoanal ultrasound. (**a**, **b**) Anterior combined internal and external anal sphincter damage due to childbirth trauma

occult sphincter defects on EAUS. Using EAUS, Donnelly et al. [3] found anal sphincter injury in 35 % of primiparous vaginal deliveries. Sultan et al. [7] reviewed EAUS findings in 79 primiparous women before and after vaginal delivery, and identified anal sphincter defects in 28 (35 %), of whom 9 (32 %) reported altered continence to stool. Sphincter defects were not identified in those women who delivered by cesarean section. Deen et al. [13] studied 46 patients with postpartum FI and found that 87 % had a recognizable anal sphincter defect on EAUS. In a prospective study, de Parades et al. [6] did not confirm previous observations that anal sphincter injury is common after forceps delivery. In a large population of 93 healthy females, anal sphincter injury was identified by ultrasonography in <13 % of cases after forceps delivery, and the development of FI was not related to these defects. The only factor with significant predictive value for anal sphincter injury was perineal tear. Pinta et al. [43] analyzed possible risk factors associated with sphincter rupture during vaginal delivery. A total of 52 females with a third-fourth degree perineal laceration were compared with 51 primiparous females with no clinically detectable perineal laceration. EAUS found a persistent defect of the EAS in 39 females (75 %) in the rupture group, compared with ten females (20 %) in the control group ($P<0.001$). An abnormal presentation was the only risk factor for anal sphincter rupture during vaginal delivery.

High-resolution multiplanar ultrasonography may help to detect sphincter damage. Three-dimensional reconstruction offers the possibility of measuring EAS length, thickness, area and volume (Fig. 5.8) [8–11]. The relationship between the radial angle and the longitudinal extent of a sphincter tear can be assessed and graded. The length of the remaining intact sphincter muscle can also be evaluated, improving the selection of patients for surgical repair of the anal sphincter complex and helping the surgeon to judge how far the repair should extend. Using multiplanar EAUS, two scoring systems have been proposed to define the severity of the sphincter damage. Starck et al. [44] introduced a specific score, with 0 indicating no

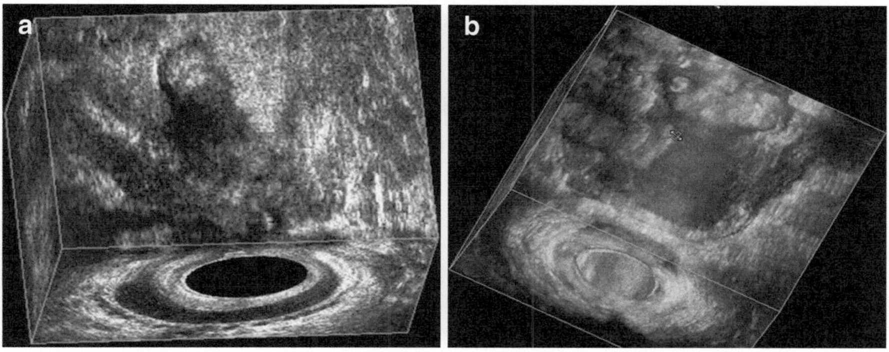

Fig. 5.8 3D endoanal ultrasound. Anterior combined internal and external anal sphincter lesion due to childbirth trauma. On the reconstructed coronal plane, the damage involves the full length of the anal canal in (**a**) and the superior 2/3 in (**b**)

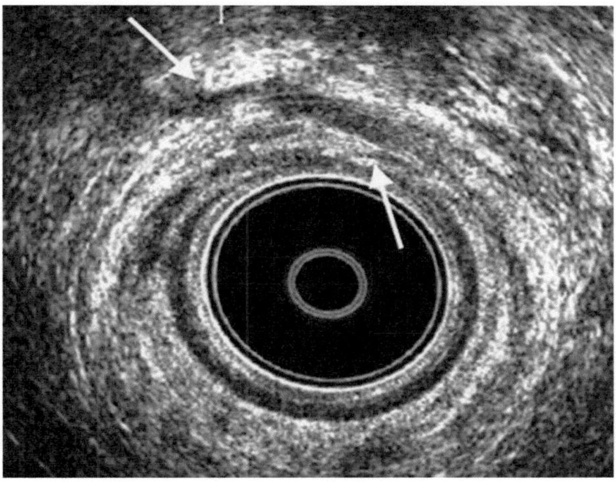

Fig. 5.9 Endoanal ultrasound. Anterior sphincter repair by overlapping (*arrows* indicate the two arms of the external sphincter)

defect and 16 corresponding to a defect >180° involving the whole length and depth of the sphincters. Recently, Noderval et al. [45] reported a simplified system for analyzing defects, including fewer categories than the Starck score and not recording partial defects of the IAS. A maximal score of 7 denotes defects in both the EAS and the IAS exceeding 90° in the axial plane and involving more than half of the sphincter length. Both systems showed good intraobserver and interoberver agreement in classifying anal sphincter defects.

Ultrasonographic imaging is useful to evaluate the result of treatments. Primary repair is usually performed within 24 h of delivery; the primary end-to-end repair is carried out by the majority of obstetricians and the alternative is an overlapping repair (Fig. 5.9) [46, 47]. However, at one year follow-up, fecal urgency, FI, and perineal pain are more common in those undergoing end-to-end repair [48]. The incidence of residual anal sphincter damage on EAUS is comparable between the two techniques. In general, a sphincter defect that exceeds 3 h on the clock face or 90° (as identified by EAUS) could make overlapping technically difficult and place the repair under tension. However, a direct relationship between size of the tear and degree of dysfunction could not be confirmed [49]. Starck et al. [50] reported that the extent of endosonographic EAS defects after primary repair of obstetric sphincter tears increased over time and was related to FI. Scheer et al. [41] demonstrated the value of EAUS and manometry in counselling women who previously sustained obstetric tears. Based on specific selection criteria, the majority of women delivered vaginally without deterioration in anal sphincter morphology and function or quality of life. Savoye-Collet et al. [51] noted improvement in FI in 86 % of patients in whom EAUS documented closure of the EAS defect after anterior sphincter repair. In contrast, patients who had a persistent defect in the EAS still had significant FI. Dobben et al. [52] also found that patients with a persistent ultrasonographic EAS defect had a worse clinical outcome than those without an EAS defect. Soerensen et al. [53] assessed the long-term function and morphology of the anal sphincters and the pelvic floor after primary repair of third or fourth degrees obstetric anal sphincter injury. At a mean follow-up of 23.7 years, cases with recurrence of FI had a significantly shorter anterior EAS length compared to controls (patients repaired and still continent) when evaluated by 3D-EAUS (8.6 vs. 10.2 mm; $p=0.03$). Functionally, anterior sphincter length correlated with increased severity of incontinence. Using 3D-EAUS, de la Portilla et al. [54] demonstrated that all the implants of silicone to treat FI were properly located in the intersphincteric space 3 months after injection. At 24 months, 75 % of implants were still properly located. They found that the continence deterioration suffered by most patients after the first year from the injection was not related to the localization and number of implants the patient had.

5.3.2 Levator Ani Injuries

Levator avulsion is the disconnection of the muscle from its insertion on the inferior pubic ramus and the pelvic sidewall, whereas tears may occur in any part of the muscle. Avulsion is a common consequence of overstretching of the LA during the second stage of labor and occurs in 10–36 % of women at the time of their first delivery [17, 18]. It is usually occult, but it has been demonstrated in delivery suite in patients with large vaginal tears. Levator avulsion, although palpable, is more accurately detected by imaging, as the lateral attachments of the LA to the pubic bone are clearly visualized. 3D-EVUS (Fig. 5.10) [27–30] and 3D-TPUS (Fig. 5.11) [19, 20] may be utilized to document major levator trauma, as can MRI [17, 18]. The defects are usually most clearly visualized on maximal PFMC. Tomographic ultrasound imaging is particularly useful [19]. A hiatal enlargement to over 25 cm^2 on Valsalva maneuver is defined as “ballooning” [55].

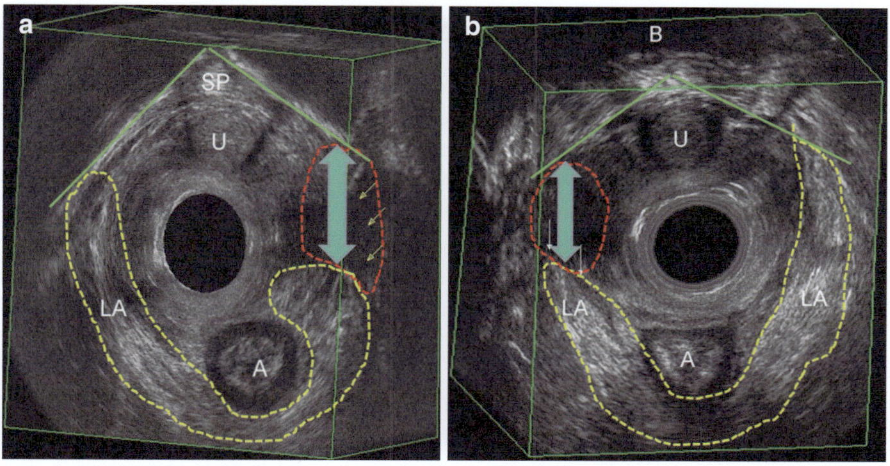

Fig. 5.10 3D endovaginal ultrasound. Levator ani (*LA*) (*arrows*) avulsion from the left inferior pubic rami in (**a**) and from the right inferior pubic rami in (**b**). *A* Anal canal, *B* bladder, *SP* symphysis pubis, *U* urethra

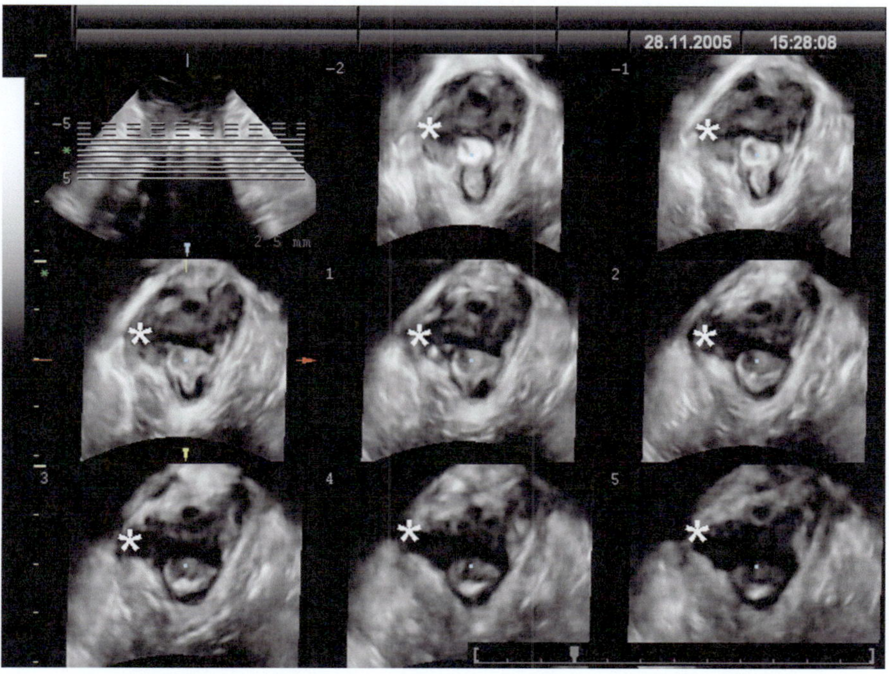

Fig. 5.11 Tomographic 3D transperineal ultrasound showing a levator ani damage avulsion from (*asterisks*) the right inferior pubic rami. (Courtesy of HP Dietz) and (from Santoro GA, Wieczorek AP, Bartram CI (eds) Pelvic floor disorders. Springer-Verlag Italia, Milan. With permission)

5.3.3 Perineal Body Damage

The perineal body plays an important role in supporting the pelvic floor and the posterior vaginal wall. This structure, through the fusion with the vagina ventrally, the perineal membrane laterally, the external anal sphincter (EAS) dorsally, forms a boundary that prevents forward and downward movement of posterior compartment [36]. Damage to the PB from obstetrical trauma may be a cause of lateral displacement of the perineal membrane and because the levator ani muscle is fused with these structures this would result in widening of the urogenital hiatus seen in women with prolapse [36]. Ultrasonography has already been used to assess the integrity of the PB, however, the current 2D-US techniques are limited in resolution of fine details and only show parts of the structures involved [56–58]. As reported by Orno et al. [59], perineal muscles cannot be visualized in their entirety by using 2D-EVUS because they originate from the walls of the pelvis and converge at the PB from different angles. Three-dimensional US imaging has the potential to overcome this limit as reported by Wagenlehner et al. [36], who found that in females with third-degree rectocele, the PB appears as two separated structures angulated downward and laterally, attached like a hinge to the posterior surface of the descending pubic ramus by the deep transverse perinei muscle (Fig. 5.12).

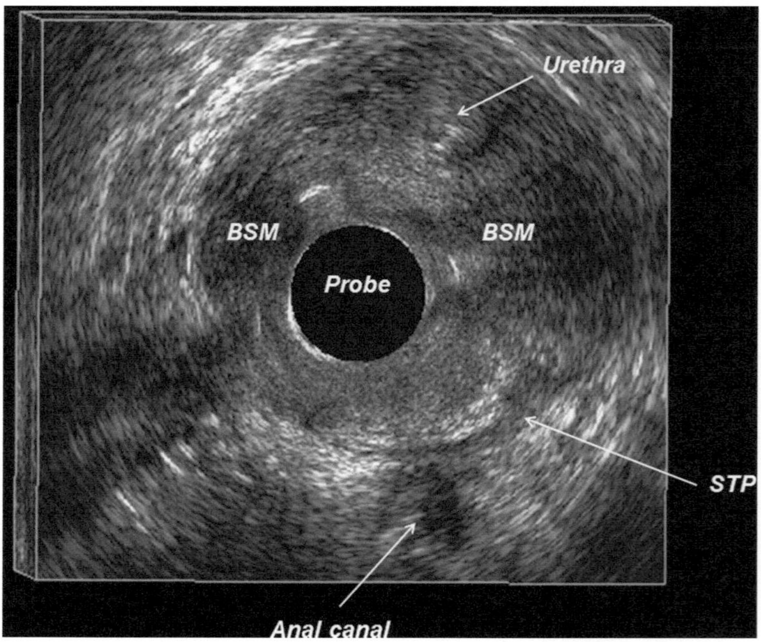

Fig. 5.12 Perineal body damage due to obstetric trauma. 3D endovaginal ultrasound cannot visualize the perineal body in the central perineum neither the superficial transverse perinei (*STP*) muscle on the right side. *BSM* Bulbospongiosus muscle

5.4 Clinical Relevance of Echographic Assessment

A meta-analysis revealed a rate of 11–15 % of FI in the general population, although it may perhaps be underestimated [42]. Intact musculature including the PR, IAS, and EAS are prerequisites for fecal control, as is a functioning nerve supply to these muscles. Other factors contributing to FI include stool consistency, rectal sensitivity and capacity, and anorectal angle. Any impairment to one or more of these factors may result in FI. Anal sphincter defects and pudendal nerve injury can occur during vaginal delivery and are by far the most common causes of FI, consequently making this problem more prevalent in women [1–7]. In patients with FI, therefore, it is fundamental to establish the underlying pathophysiology in order to choose the appropriate therapy (dietary or medications, biofeedback, sphincter repair, artificial bowel sphincter, graciloplasty, sacral nerve stimulation, injection of bulking agents) [1]. In patients with FI, EAUS has been recommended as the gold standard investigation to identify anal sphincter injury by the International Urogynecological Association (IUGA)/International Continence Society (ICS) joint report [60] and more recently by the International Consultation on Incontinence (ICI) [61]. In evaluating the role of EAUS in the management of PFD, Groenendijk et al. [62] reported that the assigned value of this modality increased significantly in cases of FI (assigned diagnostic value 68 % vs. overall value 38 %). A major impact of EAUS has been to image tears of the sphincters that are not apparent on clinical examination. Diagnosis of undetected "occult" defects may have a role in the prevention of FI, enabling a recommendation that woman at increased risk have an elective cesarean section [12, 63]. However, finding a sphincter defect does not necessarily mean that it will cause FI, as many people have sphincter lesions without having symptoms of incontinence. On the other hand, patients with FI and an apparent intact sphincter can have muscle degeneration, atrophy, or pudendal neuropathy [64]. Several studies have compared the diagnostic accuracy of EAUS and endoanal or external phased array MRI in assessing anal sphincter integrity. The current consensus is that both techniques can be used for demonstrating defects of the anal sphincter complex and can be considered useful in the selection of patients for surgery [16].

3D-TPUS has also been used to demonstrate the morphological characteristics and normal biometry of the anal sphincter complex 49 and to detect anatomical defects [65–67]. An advantage of the transperineal approach over the endoanal approach is that it avoids distortion of the anal canal by the endoluminal transducer, leading to artifactual changes in measurements. However, with TPUS, an excessive pressure applied by the transducer on the perineum or an inappropriate angle of incidence of the ultrasound beam to the anal canal may also lead to erroneous results. Compared to the 3D-EAUS, 3D-TPUS is neither able to identify clearly the conjoined longitudinal layer, the superficial transverse perinei muscle nor measure the anterior longitudinal length of EAS, and it has not been recommended by the guidelines of the International Consultation on Incontinence [61].

The functional and anatomical consequences of LA avulsion are considerable, with a reduction in muscle strength of about 1/3 and a marked alteration in anatomy [17, 19]. The main effect of avulsion is probably due to enlargement of the LH, but avulsion may also be a marker for other forms of trauma, such as damage to connective supportive structures (uterosacral ligaments, endopelvic and pubocervical fascia) that are currently difficult to detect by imaging. An enlarged LH, whether congenital, due to irreversible over-distension, or to avulsion injury, may result in excessive loading of ligamentous and fascial structures, which may, over time, lead to connective tissue failure and the development of prolapse [17]. The role of "ballooning" is likely to be much more complex than that of avulsion, and it is not clear how much of this is primary, i.e., causative, or just secondary to POP [55]. DeLancey [17] found that women with POP have an odds ratio of 7.3 for having a major levator injury compared with asymptomatic women. This data was confirmed in a larger series using TPUS [19]. Patients with an LA defect are 2.3 times more likely to have a significant cystocele, and four times as likely to have uterine prolapse. It seems that trauma to the PR component of the LA is most significant in affecting the size of the hiatus as well as symptoms and signs of prolapse [30, 68]. However, even in the absence of a levator avulsion, there are many women with highly abnormal functional anatomy of the LA. Athanasiou et al. [69] reported that LH area, measured with 2D-EVUS, was significantly larger in women with prolapse compared with those without (17.8 cm^2 vs. 13.5 cm^2). The higher the prolapse stage, the larger the hiatal area ($P<0.001$), as assessed by the maximum descent of the leading organ. Not surprisingly, this relationship is even stronger on Valsalva. 3D-EVUS may also be used to evaluate patient after PR repair with autologous fascia lata [70].

In conclusion, an integrated multicompartmental ultrasonographic approach with different modalities [31] provides a comprehensive assessment of pelvic floor damages related to childbirth and has been included in the guidelines of the International Consultation on Incontinence [71].

Index List

Anal canal
Anorectal junction
External anal sphincter
Endoanal ultrasonography
Endopelvic fascia
Endovaginal ultrasonography
Fecal incontinence
Internal anal sphincter
Intersphincteric space
Levator ani
Levator hiatus
Longitudinal muscle
Obstructed defecation
Pelvic floor disorders
Pelvic organ prolapse
Perineal body

Puboanalis muscle
Puborectalis muscle
Three-dimensional ultrasonography
Transperineal ultrasonography
Transverse perinei muscle
Uterosacral ligament

References

1. Dudding TC, Vaizey CJ, Kamm MA (2008) Obstetric anal sphincter injury. Incidence, risk factors, and management. Ann Surg 247:224–237
2. Fitzpatrick M, O'Herlihy C (2001) The effects of labour and delivery on the pelvic floor. Best Pract Res Clin Obstet Gynaecol 15:63–79
3. Donnelly V, Fynes M, Campbell D et al (1998) Obstetric events leading to anal sphincter damage. Obstet Gynecol 92:955–961
4. Minini G, Zanelli S, Inselvini P et al (2010) Mechanisms of pelvic floor trauma during vaginal delivery. In: Santoro GA, Wieczorek AP, Bartram CI (eds) Pelvic floor disorders. Springer-Verlag Italia, Milan, pp 137–141
5. Hudelist G, Gelle'n J, Singer C et al (2005) Factors predicting severe perineal trauma during childbirth: role of forceps delivery routinely combined with mediolateral episiotomy. Am J Obstet Gynecol 192:875–881
6. de Parades V, Etienney I, Thabut D et al (2004) Anal sphincter injury after forceps delivery: myth or reality? A prospective ultrasound study of 93 females. Dis Colon Rectum 47:24–34
7. Sultan AH, Kamm MA, Hudson CN et al (1993) Anal sphincter disruption during vaginal delivery. N Engl J Med 329:1905–1911
8. Di Falco G (2010) Three-dimensional endoluminal ultrasonography. In: Santoro GA, Wieczorek AP, Bartram CI (eds) Pelvic floor disorders. Springer-Verlag Italia, Milan, pp 285–295
9. Cazemier M, Terra MP, Stoker J et al (2006) Atrophy and defects detection of the external anal sphincter: comparison between three-dimensional anal endosonography and endoanal magnetic resonance imaging. Dis Colon Rectum 49:20–27
10. Williams AB, Bartram CI, Halligan S (2002) Alteration of anal sphincter morphology following vaginal delivery revealed by multiplanar anal endosonography. BJOG 109:942–946
11. Williams AB, Spencer JD, Bartram CI (2002) Assessment of third degree tears using three dimensional anal endosonography with combined anal manometry: a novel technique. BJOG 109:833–835
12. Johnson JK, Lindow SW, Duthie GS (2007) The prevalence of occult obstetric anal sphincter injury following childbirth – literature review. J Matern Fetal Neonatal Med 20:547–554
13. Deen KJ, Kumar D, Williams JG et al (1993) The prevalence of anal sphincter defects in fecal incontinence. A prospective endosonic study. Gut 34:685–688
14. Oberwalder M, Dinnewitzer A, Baig MK et al (2004) The association between late-onset fecal incontinence and obstetric anal sphincter defects. Arch Surg 139:429–432
15. Stoker J (2010) Magnetic resonance imaging. In: Santoro GA, Wieczorek AP, Bartram CI (eds) Pelvic floor disorders. Springer-Verlag Italia, Milan, pp 305–311
16. Dobben AC, Terra MP, Slors JFM et al (2007) External anal sphincter defects in patients with fecal incontinence: comparison of endoanal MR imaging and endoanal US. Radiology 242:463–471
17. DeLancey JO, Kearney R, Chou Q, Speights S, Binno S (2003) The appearance of levator ani muscle abnormalities in magnetic resonance images after vaginal delivery. Obstet Gynecol 101:46–53

18. Lien KC, Mooney B, DeLancey JO, Ashton-Miller JA (2004) Levator ani muscle stretch induced by simulated vaginal birth. Obstet Gynecol 103:31–40
19. Dietz H (2007) Quantification of major morphological abnormalities of the levator ani. Ultrasound Obstet Gynecol 29:329–334
20. Dietz H, Gillespie A, Phadke P (2007) Avulsion of the pubovisceral muscle associated with large vaginal tear after normal vaginal delivery at term. Aust N Z J Obstet Gynaecol 47:341–344
21. Dietz HP (2004) Ultrasound imaging of the pelvic floor. Part II: three-dimensional aspects. Ultrasound Obstet Gynecol 23:615–625
22. Dietz H, Shek K (2008) Levator avulsion and grading of pelvic floor muscle strength. Int Urogynecol J Pelvic Floor Dysfunct 19:633–636
23. Albrich S, Laterza R, Skala C, Salvatore S, Koelbl H, Naumann G (2012) Impact of mode of delivery on levator morphology: a prospective observational study with three-dimensional ultrasound early in the postpartum period. BJOG 119:51–61
24. Cassadò Garriga J, Pessarrodona Isern A, Espuna Pons M et al (2011) Four-dimensional sonographic evaluation of avulsion of the levator ani according to delivery mode. Ultrasound Obstet Gynecol 38:701–706
25. Cassadò Garriga J, Pessarrodona Isern A, Espuna Pons M et al (2011) Tridimensional sonographic anatomical changes on pelvic floor muscle according to the type of delivery. Int Urogynecol J Pelvic Floor Dysfunct 22:1011–1018
26. Rostaminia G, White D, Quiroz LH, Shobeiri SA (2014) 3D pelvic floor ultrasound findings and severity of anal incontinence. Int Urogynecol J Pelvic Floor Dysfunct 25:623–629
27. van Delft K, Thakar R, Sultan A, Schwertner-Tiepelmann N, Kluivers K (2014) Levator ani muscle avulsion during childbirth: a risk prediction model. BJOG 121:1155–1163
28. van Delft K, Thakar R, Shobeiri SA, Sultan AH (2014) Levator hematoma at the attachment zone as an early marker for levator ani muscle avulsion. Ultrasound Obstet Gynecol 43:210–217
29. van Delft K, Sultan AH, Thakar R, Schwertner-Tiepelmann N, Kluivers K (2014) The relationship between postpartum levator ani muscle avulsion and signs and symptoms of pelvic floor dysfunction. BJOG 121:1164–1172
30. Rostaminia G, White D, Hegde A, Quiroz LH, Davila GW, Shobeiri SA (2013) Levator ani deficiency and pelvic organ prolapse severity. Obstet Gynecol 121:1017–1024
31. Santoro GA, Wieczorek AP, Dietz HP et al (2011) State of the art: an integrated approach to pelvic floor ultrasonography. Ultrasound Obstet Gynecol 37:381–396
32. Dietz HP (2004) Ultrasound imaging of the pelvic floor. Part I: two-dimensional aspects. Ultrasound Obstet Gynecol 23:80–92
33. Braekken IH, Majida M, Ellstrom-Engh M, Dietz HP, Umek W, Bo K (2008) Test-retest and intra-observer repeatability of two-, three- and four-dimensional perineal ultrasound of pelvic floor muscle anatomy and function. Int Urogynecol J Pelvic Floor Dysfunct 19:227–235
34. Santoro GA, Wieczorek AP, Stankiewicz A, Wozniak MM, Bogusiewicz M, Rechbereger T (2009) High-resolution three dimensional endovaginal ultrasonography in the assessment of pelvic floor anatomy: a preliminary study. Int Urogynecol J Pelvic Floor Dysfunct 20: 1213–1222
35. Santoro GA, Wieczorek AP, Shobeiri SA et al (2011) Interobserver and interdisciplinary reproducibility of 3D endovaginal ultrasound assessment of pelvic floor anatomy. Int Urogynecol J Pelvic Floor Dysfunct 22:53–59
36. Wagenlehner FME, Del Amo E, Santoro GA, Petros PE (2013) Live anatomy of the perineal body in patients with 3rd degree rectocele. Colorectal Dis 15:1416–1422
37. Santoro GA, Fortling B (2007) The advantages of volume rendering in three-dimensional endosonography of the anorectum. Dis Colon Rectum 50:359–368
38. Santoro GA, Di Falco G (2010) Endoanal and endorectal ultrasonography: methodology and normal pelvic floor anatomy. In: Santoro GA, Wieczorek AP, Bartram CI (eds) Pelvic floor disorders. Springer-Verlag Italia, Milan, pp 91–102
39. Regadas FSP, Murad-Regadas SM, Lima DMR et al (2007) Anal canal anatomy showed by three-dimensional anorectal ultrasonography. Surg Endosc 21:2207–2211

40. Roos AM, Thakar R, Sultan AH (2010) Outcome of primary repair of obstetric anal sphincter injuries (OASIS): does the grade of tear matter? Ultrasound Obstet Gynecol 36:368–374
41. Scheer I, Thakar R, Sultan AH (2009) Mode of delivery after previous obstetric anal sphincter injuries (OASIS)–a reappraisal? Int Urogynecol J Pelvic Floor Dysfunct 20:1095–1101
42. Oberwalder M, Connor J, Wexner SD (2003) Meta-analysis to determine the incidence of obstetric anal sphincter damage. Br J Surg 90:1333–1337
43. Pinta TM, Kylanpaa ML, Teramo KAW, Luukkonen PS (2004) Sphincter rupture and anal incontinence after first vaginal delivery. Acta Obstet Gynecol Scand 83:917–922
44. Starck M, Bohe M, Valentin L (2003) Results of endosonographic imaging of the anal sphincter 2–7 days after primary repair of third or fourth-degree obstetric sphincter tears. Ultrasound Obstet Gynecol 22:609–615
45. Norderval S, Dehli T, Vonen B (2009) Three-dimensional endoanal ultrasonography: intraobserver and interobserver agreement using scoring systems for classification of anal sphincter defects. Ultrasound Obstet Gynecol 33:337–343
46. Fernando RJ, Sultan AH, Kettle C et al (2006) Repair techniques for obstetric anal sphincter injuries: a randomized controlled trial. Obstet Gynecol 107:1261–1268
47. Sultan AH, Monga AK, Kumar D et al (1999) Primary repair of obstetric anal sphincter rupture using the overlap technique. Br J Obstet Gynaecol 106:318–323
48. Malouf AJ, Norton CS, Engel AF, Nicholls RJ, Kamm MA (2000) Long term results of overlapping anterior anal-sphincter repair for obstetric trauma. Lancet 355:260–265
49. Voyvodic F, Rieger NA, Skinner S et al (2003) Endosonographic imaging of anal sphincter injury. Does the size of the tear correlate with the degree of dysfunction? Dis Colon Rectum 46:735–741
50. Starck M, Bohe M, Valentin L (2006) The extent of endosonographic anal sphincter defects after primary repair of obstetric sphincter tear increases over time and is related to anal incontinence. Ultrasound Obstet Gynecol 27:188–197
51. Savoye-Collet C, Savoye G, Koning E et al (1999) Anal endosonography after sphincter repair: specific patterns related to clinical outcome. Abdom Imaging 24:569–573
52. Dobben AC, Terra MP, Deutekom M (2007) The role of endoluminal imaging in clinical outcome of overlapping anterior anal sphincter repair in patients with fecal incontinence. AJR Am J Roentgenol 189:70–77
53. Soerensen MM, Pedersen BG, Santoro GA, Buntzen S, Bek K, Laurberg S (2014) Long-term function and morphology of the anal sphincters and the pelvic floor after primary repair of obstetric anal sphincter injury. Colorectal Dis 16(10):O347–O355
54. de la Portilla F, Vega J, Rada R et al (2009) Evaluation by three-dimensional anal endosonography of injectable silicone biomaterial (PTQ) implants to treat fecal incontinence: long-term localization and relation with the deterioration of the continence. Tech Coloproctol 13: 195–199
55. Shek K, Dietz H (2009) The effect of childbirth on hiatal dimensions: a prospective observational study. Obstet Gynecol 113:1272–1278
56. Zetterstrom JP, Mellgren A, Madoff RD, Kim DG, Wong WD (1998) Perineal body measurement improves evaluation of anterior sphincter lesions during enodoanal ultrasonography. Dis Colon Rectum 41:705–713
57. Dietz HP, Steensma AB (2005) Posterior compartment prolapse on two-dimensional and three dimensional pelvic floor ultrasound: the distinction between true rectocele, perineal hypermobility and enterocele. Ultrasound Obstet Gynecol 26:73–77
58. Oberwalder M, Thaler K, Baig MK et al (2004) Anal ultrasound and endosonographic measurement of perineal body thickness: a new evaluation for fecal incontinence in females. Surg Endosc 18:650–654
59. Orn AK, Marsal K, Herbst A (2008) Ultrasonographic anatomy of perineal structures during pregnancy and immediately following obstetric injury. Ultrasound Obstet Gynecol 32:527–534
60. Haylen BT, de Ridder D, Freeman RM et al (2010) An international urogynecological association (IUGA)/international continence society (ICS) joint report on the terminology for female pelvic floor dysfunction. Int Urogynecol J Pelvic Floor Dysfunct 21:5–26

61. Bliss DZ, Mellgren A, Whitehead WE et al (2013). Chapter 16. Assessment and conservative management of faecal incontinence and quality of life in adults. In: Abrams P, Cardozo L, Khoury S, Wein A (eds) 5th International Consultation on Incontinence. pp 1443–1486
62. Groenendijk AG, Birnie E, de Blok S et al (2009) Clinical-decision taking in primary pelvic organ prolapse; the effects of diagnostic tests on treatment selection in comparison with a consensus meeting. Int Urogynecol J Pelvic Floor Dysfunct 20:711–719
63. Andrews V, Sultan A, Thakar R, Jones P (2006) Occult anal sphincter injuries—myth or reality? BJOG 113:195–200
64. Vaizey CJ, Kamm MA, Bartram CI (1997) Primary degeneration of the internal anal sphincter as a cause of passive faecal incontinence. Lancet 349:612–615
65. Huang WC, Yang SH, Yang JM (2007) Three-dimensional transperineal sonographic characteristics of the anal sphincter complex in nulliparous women. Ultrasound Obstet Gynecol 30:210–220
66. Yagel S, Valsky DV (2006) Three-dimensional transperineal ultrasonography for evaluation of the anal sphincter complex: another dimension in understanding peripartum sphincter trauma. Ultrasound Obstet Gynecol 27:119–123
67. Weinstein MM, Pretorius DH, Jung SAI, Nager CW, Mittal RK (2009) Transperineal 3-dimensional ultrasound imaging for detection of anatomical defects in the anal sphincter complex muscles. Clin Gastroenterol Hepatol 7:205–211
68. DeLancey JO, Morgan DM, Fenner DE et al (2007) Comparison of levator ani muscle defects and function in women with and without pelvic organ prolapse. Obstet Gynecol 109:295–302
69. Athanasiou S, Chaliha C, Toozs-Hobson P, Salvatore S, Khullar V, Cardozo L (2007) Direct imaging of the pelvic floor muscles using two-dimensional ultrasound: a comparison of women with urogenital prolapse versus controls. BJOG 114:882–888
70. Rostaminia G, Shobeiri SA, Quiroz LH (2013) Surgical repair of bilateral levator ani muscles with ultrasound guidance. Int Urogynecol J Pelvic Floor Dysfunct 24:1237–1239
71. Tubaro A, Vodušek DB, Amarenco G et al (2013). Chapter 7. Imaging, neurophysiological testing and other tests. In: Abrams P, Cardozo L, Khoury S, Wein A (eds). 5th International Consultation on Incontinence. pp 507–622

Combined Three-Dimensional Transperineal Ultrasonography (3-D TPUS) and Magnetic Resonance Imaging (MRI) After Vaginal Delivery

6

Vittorio L. Piloni and Fabio Muggia

6.1 Introduction

Childbirth is the most common cause of direct injury to the vaginal tube, its muscular support and, occasionally, to the anal sphincter complex as a result of the pressure exerted during the passage of the infant's head [1]. A large number of variables may account for damage to the pelvic floor, including precipitous labor with sudden descent of the infant and expulsion of the head, abnormal presentation necessitating difficult forceps extraction, large size of the baby [2], unusually friable maternal tissues, etc., all of which being more common and extensive in primiparous women. Using a mathematical model, Lien et al. [3] have demonstrated that during the second stage of labor the largest stretch ratio, defined as the tissue length under stretch divided by the original tissue length, does occur in the medial pubococcygeus muscle which is the shortest, most medial, and ventral portion of the levator ani muscle, thus leading to an approximately four times increase of the initial levator hiatus diameter. Conversely, the iliococcygeus muscle, which lies on a higher plane, is more prone to being stretched during the first stage of labor. While severe vaginal and perineal lacerations are usually easily recognized and promptly repaired, more subtle changes are frequently overlooked at the time of delivery and go undetected until pelvic floor weakness or anal sphincter derangement develop later as result of new deliveries, superimposed anorectal or pelvic surgery, menopause, and aging.

V.L. Piloni (✉)
Diagnostic Imaging Centre, Villa Igea Clinic,
Via Maggini 200, Ancona, 30127, Italy
e-mail: vittorio.piloni@libero.it

F. Muggia
Centro di Medicina Spa,
Viale della Repubblica 10/b, Villorba (TV), 31050, Italy
e-mail: fabiomuggia@libero.it, dorrotfabiomuggia@fabiomuggia.com

D. Riva, G. Minini (eds.), *Childbirth-Related Pelvic Floor Dysfunction: Risk Factors, Prevention, Evaluation, and Treatment*,
DOI 10.1007/978-3-319-18197-4_6

On the other hand, connective tissue healing and recovery of muscular tonic activity have also been demonstrated to occur after just 7 months from delivery [4] leading to the hypothesis that the bulk of recovery takes place in the early postpartum period [5]. With the exception of anal endosonography, which is considered the gold standard for quantification of anal sphincter defects and prediction of fecal incontinence [6–11], other available imaging techniques have not extensively been considered until the advent of three-dimensional transperineal ultrasonography (3-D TPUS) and fast magnetic resonance imaging (MRI) [12–14]. Bulking evidence does exist in the literature today to state that using them is of unique value in both the postdelivery period and subsequent years for recognition of unknown changes which, if undetected, will eventually lead to the development of pelvic organ prolapse, rectocele [15] and even double incontinence. In this chapter, the basic principles, diagnostic criteria, and clinical application of 3-D TPUS and MRI following parturition will be described. In addition, a combined approach which has been given the name of "Integrated Fusion Imaging Protocol" (IFIP) is presented for routine application after vaginal delivery in the clinical practice. More precisely, while a judicious policy combining 3-D TPUS and static MRI is the preferred approach in the early postdelivery period (i.e., within 2 weeks) so as to avoid additional stress to the damaged maternal tissues, a dynamic MRI study including the Valsalva maneuver and also the expulsion of rectal contrast is better suited later (within 6 months), leaving to dynamic 2-D TPUS the main role of diagnostic tool in the follow-up period (fourth-to-sixth decade). This strategy is suitable (1) to recognize and repair promptly most severe changes and (2) to unveil occult lesions and prevent them from evolving in overt pelvic floor dysfunctions at a later age.

6.2 Imaging Modalities

6.2.1 Three-Dimensional Transperineal Sonography

Given the limited availability of anal endosonography among gynecologists and superior familiarity with the intralabial approach by either two-dimensional or, more recently, 3-D TPS, the latter technique has rapidly gained wide acceptance all over the world. In the clinical practice, following optimal standardization of the technique by Dietz et al. [16], the examination has become the preferred imaging modality to assess pelvic floor anatomy after vaginal delivery today. The following is a description of the technical principles, diagnostic criteria, and practical application of 3-D TPS for the evaluation of most common childbirth-induced injuries.

6.2.1.1 Imaging Technique

Without any interference with normal movement of pelvic organs (as occurs when using intracavitary transducers), modern 3-D pelvic floor ultrasonography allows motorized acquisition, reconstruction, and analysis of a volume dataset which include measurement of distances and areas of pelvic structures involved in vaginal delivery. Currently available 3-D probes combine an electronic curved array of

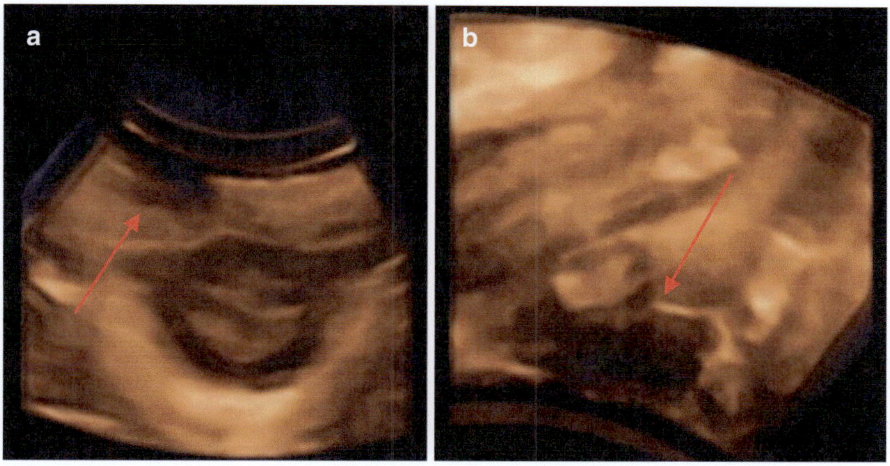

Fig. 6.1 3-D rendering of anal sphincter complex performed 1 week after vaginal delivery with image display on the axial (**a**) and sagittal (**b**) plane: *arrows* point to a hypoechoic defect of the external anal sphincter located at the 11 o'clock position

3–8 MHz with mechanical sector technology allowing fast motorized sweeps along an acquisition angle of 70°, through an arch of 85° wide enough to include in the frame both branches of the pubococcygeal muscle. All the sonographer needs is to maintain the probe in position during image acquisition that takes approximately 1–2 s to complete. Thereafter, volume datasets are stored on a separate server and assessment of all anatomic structures is permitted using tomographic or multislice imaging capability. The two basic display modes commonly used on 3-D US systems include the multiplanar or orthogonal display mode (either in the midsagittal, coronal, or axial plane), and the semitransparent representation of voxels in a region of interest also known as "rendered image" which emphasizes surfaces, soft tissues, bone and fluid-filled spaces, depending on the chosen rendering setting (Fig. 6.1). Four-dimensional (4-D) imaging is also possible implying that the real-time acquisition of volume datasets is being represented in orthogonal planes or rendered mode. The 4-D view is obtained in the same way as 3-D, but the speed of the mechanical tilting by probe crystals is faster while the spatial resolution is lower. The duration of a sequence ranges from 3–5 s to 8–10 s depending on the frame-rate and on the resolution in use. Offline postprocessing with no need for presence of the patient is also permitted, including image magnification, contrast and density adjustment, multislice view by tomographic ultrasound imaging (TUI) tool (Fig. 6.2) and measurement of established parameters. The ultrasound system in use by us is a General Electric Kretz Voluson E8 model scanner (General Electric Kretz Technik GmbH, Zipf, Austria) equipped with a 4–8 MHz multifrequency convex volumetric transducer (RAB L 8) allowing depiction of the entire genital hiatus, the right and left levator ani limbs, and the bladder neck (cranially). For the examination, the patient lies supine on the table, with her bladder half-filled after partial cleansing of distal gut. For better orientation and identification of pertinent anatomy by the

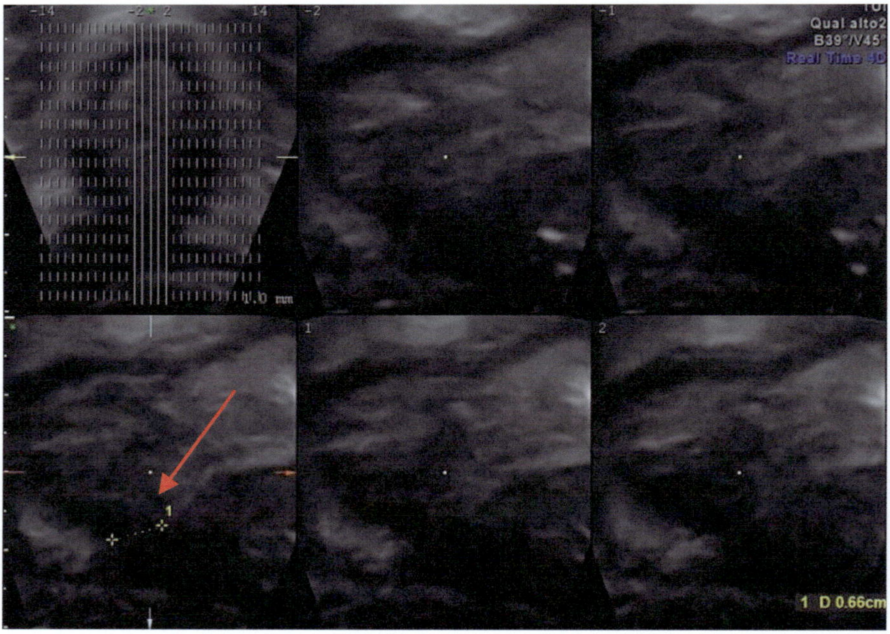

Fig. 6.2 Tomographic ultrasound imaging (TUI) of anatomic defect (*arrow*) seen on multiple midsagittal planes

examiner, image display on the screen is given up-down with acquisition starting on the midsagittal plane.

6.2.1.2 Standard Measurements

The following measurements, performed at rest or during functional tests (Kegel and Valsalva maneuver), are taken in the midsagittal plane:

- Bladder wall thickness with no more than 20 mL residue (n.v., 5 mm).
- Bladder–symphysis distance, defined as the vertical distance between the bladder neck and the horizontal line tangent to the lower margin of the symphysis pubis (n.v., no more than 1 cm above at rest and no more than 1 cm below on straining).
- The γ angle, defined as the angle between the inferior edge of the symphysis pubis and the anterior margin of the urethrovesical junction.
- The retrovesical (β) angle, defined as the angle between the proximal urethra and the trigonal surface of the bladder.
- Diameters and area of the levator hiatus in the axial plane after identification of the so-called plane of minimal hiatal dimension which extend from the posterior margin of the symphysis to the posterior anorectal junction. According to Dietz, a hiatal area exceeding 25 cm^2 is considered indicative of abnormal hiatal distensibility.

6.2.1.3 Abnormal Findings

Most common changes seen in the early post vaginal delivery period include the following:

- Gaping of the genital hiatus
- Absent or reduced ability to perform Kegel or Valsalva maneuver
- Asymmetry of the genital area
- Unilateral discontinuity of levator limb from tear or avulsion (*see* Fig. 5.1)
- Anal sphincter defect
- Fascial detachment

Medium-term (within 6 months) and long-term (after the fourth decade) changes include the following:

- Cysto-urethrocele
- Rectocele
- Enterocele
- Funneling of the bladder neck
- Vaginal vault prolapse
- Sliding of anterior or posterior vaginal wall
- Focal scarring of anterior anal canal

6.2.2 Magnetic Resonance Imaging

Thanks to the advances in technology registered during the last two decades which permit rapid image acquisition and display on any plane and to the inherent superior contrast resolution of the technique, MRI is an unsurpassed imaging modality providing unique details of postdelivery pelvic anatomy in a safe and noninvasive manner. Through this, exquisite depiction of all pelvic structures directly involved in parturition can routinely be obtained in a resting state, including the vaginal canal, levator ani muscles, anal sphincters, perineal body, endopelvic fascia, and ligaments. In addition, a dynamic series can also be acquired in the three orthogonal planes while the patient performs a Valsalva maneuver and even during emptying her bladder and/or rectal ampulla [17].

6.2.2.1 Imaging Technique

Postpartum MR scans of the pelvis are usually taken early (within 2 weeks) and late (within 6 months) after delivery with the patient supine using a 1.5-T superconducting conventional (horizontal) magnet system (Philips Medical System, Achieva model, The Netherlands) equipped with high-speed gradients and a surface phased-array coil (Body SENSE XL Torso) wrapped around the patient's pelvis. A soft rubber catheter, 3 mm in diameter, is gently inserted within the anal canal to act as a luminal marker (early study) and for subsequent contrast administration (late study).

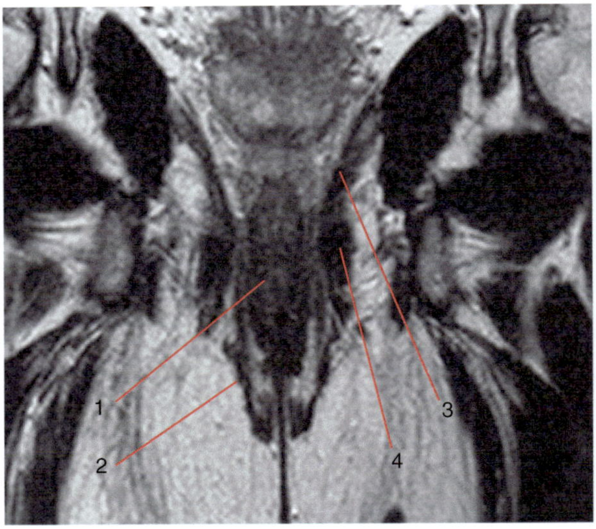

Fig. 6.3 Coronal oblique T2-weighted image of the anal sphincter complex allowing clear depiction of the internal and external anal sphincter muscle (*1, 2*) and iliococcygeal and puborectalis muscle (*3, 4*), respectively

Images are obtained in all three planes (sagittal, axial, and coronal) as different, useful information is derived from each. The typical examination is usually conducted on the following lines:

Early Study (Static Examination)

T2-weighted images are obtained first in the sagittal plane to provide a complete evaluation of pelvic floor anatomy using fast recovery spin echo pulse sequence (TR/TE, 3,704/90 ms; FA, 90°; FOV, 320 cm; BW, 253.0; slice thickness, 4 mm; interslice gap, 1 mm; matrix size, 444 × 310; ETL, 18 and 4 excitations; scan time, 2.24 min). Then, following exact localization of the intra-anal catheter, oblique axial and coronal images are taken with the same pulse sequence in a plane perpendicular and parallel to the catheter, respectively, so as to obtain true orthogonal views of the anal sphincter complex (Fig. 6.3) and contemporary differentiation of the various components of the levator ani muscle, i.e., the iliococcygeal, the pubococcygeal, and the coccygeal muscles. Occasionally, a proton density (PD) and a short tau inversion recovery (STIR) pulse sequences are also obtained for better evidence of ligaments anatomy and rule out anovaginal fistula.

Late Study (Static + Dynamic Examination)

Following the study described in 3.1.1, intrarectal injection of up to 200 mL of acoustic gel is administered and a BFFE pulse sequence (TR/TE, 2.8/1.39 ms; FA, 90°; BW, 1255.5; slice thickness, 15 mm; matrix size, 160 × 160; image update acquisition, 1/0.891 s; scan time, 48 s and two excitations) is obtained with the patient at rest and during active contraction of pelvic floor musculature (Kegel maneuver). Then, after patient coaching to start the rectal emptying at will and just make notice of it by intercom, contemporary acquisition of images is obtained by the examiner. Using the same pulse sequence, images are also acquired in the oblique coronal plane centered at the anorectal junction (ARJ) during continuous rectal emptying for evidence of any outlet obstruction and excessive rectal floor descent. Finally, the levator ani hiatus is imaged in the horizontal axial plane using a multislice technique (TR/TE, 3.1/1.5 ms; FA, 45; slice thickness, 10 mm; BW, 1041.7; matrix, 160×160; NEX, 2 excitations; N° of slices, 3–4; scan time, 14.9 s) with section planes located at the superior margin of the symphysis pubis (upper level), at its inferior margin (central level), and at the perineal body (lower level) while the patient is asked to strain maximally (Valsalva maneuver) in a steady state. A complete summary of the standard imaging protocol described above is presented in Table 6.1.

6.2.2.2 Image Analysis

Key images for interpretation of postdelivery anatomy are taken on the *axial plane* for the assessment of the levator hiatus boundaries and contents, vaginal configuration, and urethra, paraurethral, and paravaginal supporting structures (Fig. 6.4) as described by DeLancey [18]. More precisely, sections taken at the level of the uterine cervix in DeLancey level I show the fascial condensations of the uterosacral ligaments, cardinal ligaments, and round ligaments as thin linear structures of low signal intensity. Sections taken in DeLancey level II depict the female urethra as three concentric rings of different signal intensity and the normal vaginal configuration as a two-layered structure showing a typical W-shape structure. Moreover, as described by Kim et al. [19], the periurethral, paraurethral, and pubourethral ligaments are also seen as a thin hypointense structures connecting the posterior aspect of the urethra and the arcus tendineus fascia pelvis. The pubococcygeus and puborectalis muscles (visceral portion of levator ani muscle) are seen as symmetric structures of low signal intensity equal to that of the obturator muscle (OM). Finally, the sciatic nerve is seen as dark dot-shaped structure whose identification is facilitated by consistently recognizable anatomic landmarks along its course [20]. The *sagittal plane* is ideal to depict and measure the perineal body position and size relative to the pubic bone [21], together with assessment of the total vaginal length and levator plate caudal inclination according to Bump et al. [22]. The *coronal plane* displays at best the anal sphincter complex architecture together with the iliococcygeus muscle attachment to the obturator muscle via the endopelvic fascia. Dynamic MRl images are evaluated in the three orthogonal planes on straining and evacuation for assessment of pelvic organs prolapse and anorectal morphology.

6.2.2.3 Standard Measurements

- The "HMO system" as described by Comiter et al. [23] has been used since 1999 for quantification of pelvic floor relaxation and visceral descent on midsagittal images, taking (a) the H line to measure the distance from the inferior symphysis pubis to the posterior ARJ; (b) the vertical distance of pelvic organs (O) relative to the pubococcygeal line (PCL) to assess their descent ; and (c) the M line to evaluate levator plate activity by measuring the perpendicular distance from the PCL to the most distal aspect of the H line. Normal values reported for the H and M line, are 5 and 2 cm, respectively. More recently, however, in order to eliminate discrepancies between imaging and clinical assessment, the midpubic line

Table 6.1 Protocol for pelvic floor MRI after vaginal delivery by Philips Achieva scanner (1.5 T) and SENSE XL TORSO coil

Parameter	Series 1	Series 2	Series 3	Series 4	Series 5	Series 6
Study type	Static	Static	Static	Dynamic	Dynamic	Dynamic
Plane	Sagittal	Coronal oblique	Axial oblique	Mid sagittal	Mid coronal	Axial multislice
TR (ms)	4,435	3,649	4,656	2.8	2.8	3.1
TE (ms)	100	100	100	1.3	1.3	1.5
BW	253.0	172.6	252.4	1225.5	1225.5	1041.7
ETL	18	18	18	17	17	17
NEX	4	4	4	2	2	2
FOV (FH-RL-AP)	250*250*177	250*250*138	250*250*173	260*260*134	250*250*-112	250*250*112
Matrix	560 (256*246)	560 (264*270)	560 (264*270)	336 (192*181)	320 (160*153)	336 (160*153)
Slice/gap (mm)	3.70–0.13	3.5–0.35	3.5–0.35	10	10	10
Flip angle (°)	90	90	90			45
Scan time (sec)	148	148	174	48	48	14.9
Slices (n°)	20	20	20	50	50	3
Pulse sequence	FSE T2-W	FSE T2-W	FSE T2-W	BFFE	BFFE	BFFE
Fold over direction	F→H	R→L	R→L	R→L	R→L	A→P

Notes: *F* foot, *H* head, *R* right, *L* left, *A* anterior, *P* posterior, *FSE* fast spin echo, *BFFE* balance fast field echo, *T2-W* T2-weighted

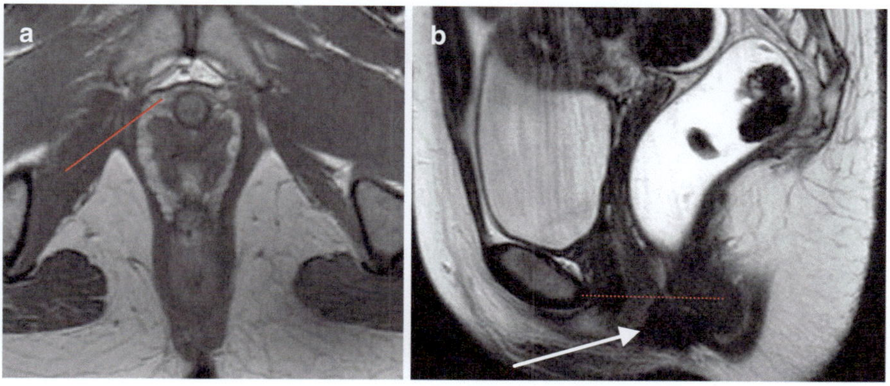

Fig. 6.4 Key images for normal MR anatomy identification on the axial (**a**) and sagittal (**b**) plane: note the aspect of the paraurethral attachments and the H-shaped vaginal configuration (**a**, *red line*); and the triangular-shaped structure with low signal intensity of the perineal body (**b**, *white arrow*). The *red dotted line* indicates the hymeneal plane

(MPL) drawn across the midsagittal aspect of the pubic bone, as described by Singh et al. [24], has been suggested as preferable reference instead of the PCL, because it is coterminous with the level of the hymeneal ring which provides a precisely identifiable landmark for reference universally adopted, as described by Bump et al. [22].

- The position of the perineal body (PB) is measured as a perpendicular line drawn between the reference line and the anterior margin of the anal sphincter muscle. This distance is assumed as an indication of the recovery of striated perineal muscles.
- The slope of levator plate angle (LPA)° is measured at rest and on straining relative to the horizontal line and considered zero when it is parallel to the reference line, negative when it is above in a clockwise direction, and positive when it is below in a counter-clockwise direction.
- The width of the levator hiatus is measured between the medial aspect of the right and left levator ani muscle at the level of the lateral vaginal wall [25] while its length is measured from the symphysis pubis to the posterior rectal wall at the ARJ.
- The characteristics of LA signal intensities are described qualitatively as being either the same, higher or lower [5] when compared to that of the obturator muscle (OM).
- The mean thickness and degree of asymmetry of the LA limbs are measured by calculating the thicker limb plus that of the thinner limb divided by 2, and the thicker limb divided by the thinner limb, respectively [19].

6.2.2.4 Abnormal Findings

Common anatomic changes reported as result of a traumatic delivery include vaginal lacerations, anal sphincter defects, levator ani avulsion and tears, perineal body disruption and descent, paravaginal and paraurethral ligament detachment, and occasional urethrovaginal fistulae. Most of them will recover within 6 months so

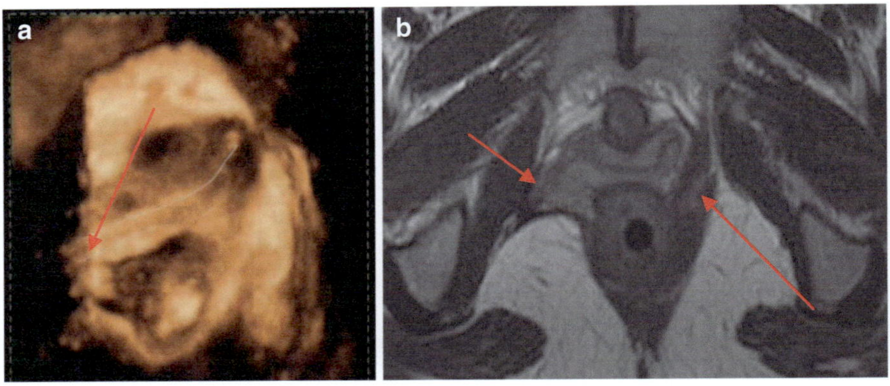

Fig. 6.5 IFIP of right pubococcygeal muscle avulsion after childbirth traumatic vaginal delivery: compared to 3-D rendering TPUS (**a**), axial MR imaging (**b**) offer better evidence of the paravaginal defect (*short arrow*) and the focal discontinuity with increased signal intensity from fibrofatty degeneration (*long arrow*) of the left hypertrophic pubococcygeal muscle

that no significant complaint will develop despite their persistence on MR imaging. From a practical point of view, they may be subdivided into morphologic changes visible in the early post-delivery study and functional changes seen at best in the late dynamic study, as follows.

Morphologic Changes

These include a variety of changes in LA signal intensity, topography and thickness due to muscular distension, ischemia, and neural trauma, and in the supporting structures, as follows:

- Loss of normal vaginal configuration and lateral shift of its posterior wall, consistent with presence of paravaginal defect
- Distortion, discontinuity, and fluttering of paraurethral supporting structures
- Discontinuity, interruption, and avulsion of unilateral or bilateral LA limbs with or without decreased thickness, asymmetry index, and higher T2 muscle signal intensity (Fig. 6.5)
- Focal defect of the anal sphincter complex
- Focal detachment of the endopelvic fascia
- PB disruption and reduced thickness
- Levator hiatus asymmetry
- Anovaginal fistula (Fig. 6.6)
- Increased signal intensity of pudendal nerve (edema)

Functional Changes

On dynamic MRI, criteria that have been used in the literature to define pelvic organ prolapse [26] include (a) bladder base descent more than 1 cm from the PCL (cystocele); (b) cervix or vaginal vault less than 1 cm above the PCL or below it (genital

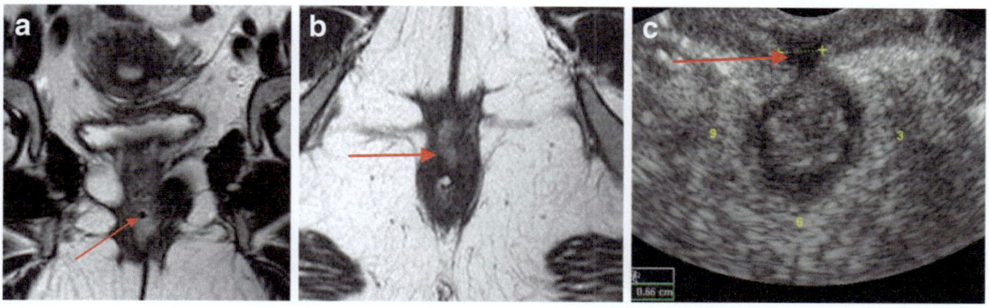

Fig. 6.6 IFIP in a 32-year-old woman with fourth degree tear, disruption of the right pubococcygeal muscle, anovaginal fistula (*arrow*), and left-sided temporary colostomy after rectal suture repair and subsequent dehiscence (**a**). Contemporary axial STIR image showing the abnormal anovaginal communication as a focal change with increased signal intensity (*arrow*, **b**), and persistent hypoechoic lesion located at 12 o'clock position seen by 2D ultrasonography (*arrow*, **c**) 6 months later

prolapse); (c) bowel between the vagina and rectum below the PCL, and the widening of the rectovaginal space or abnormal deepening of the cul-de-sac (enterocele); (d) descent of the ARJ greater than 2 cm below the PCL (rectal prolapse). In addition, rectocele is defined as an abnormal outpouching of the rectum greater than 2 cm impinging on the hymen ring. Other features associated with late functional disorders of the pelvic floor after childbirth trauma include the following:

- Involuntary loss of urine and/or intrarectal contrast (incontinence) with lack of apposition of anal walls
- Abnormal evacuation pattern, i.e., outlet obstruction, trapping in rectocele, and increased rectal floor descent
- Delayed recovery of normal PB position
- Ballooning and increased diameters of the levator hiatus with multiple organ impingement increased levator plate angle (>44°) on straining

6.3 Integrated Fusion Imaging Protocol (IFIP)

Women who delivered vaginally and had had obstetric factors commonly associated with pelvic floor injury, such as forceps or vacuum delivery, anal sphincter laceration, prolonged second stage of labor, precipitous delivery, and shoulder dystocia, are potential candidate to undergo a combined, three-step IFIP diagnostic imaging approach, as follows.

6.3.1 First Step (Within 2 Weeks)

A 3-D TPUS is firstly performed for evidence and grading of anatomic changes involving the vaginal wall, perineal muscles, levator hiatus and to rule out any defect of the anal sphincter complex by taking advantage from the tomographic

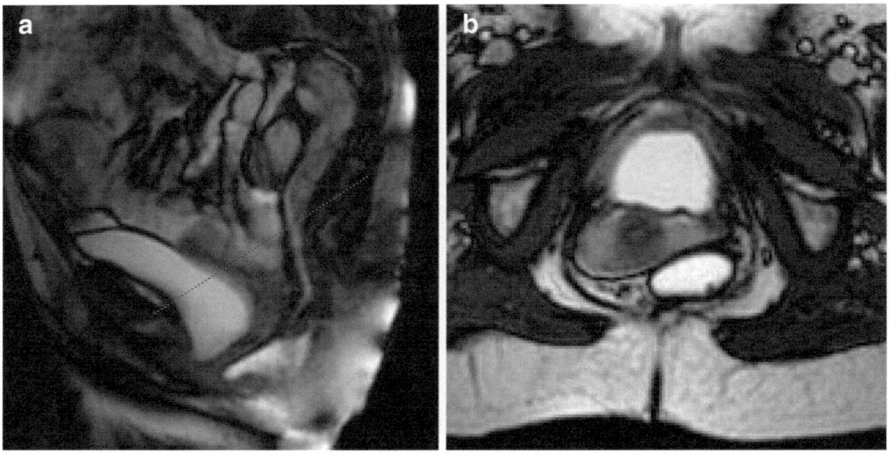

Fig. 6.7 Excessive displacement of pelvic organs with respect to the reference PCL line (*dotted line*, **a**) during evacuation of rectal contrast in a 55-year-old woman with history of four vaginal deliveries and obstructed defecation syndrome. Levator hiatus ballooning and impingement of bladder base, cervix, and distal gut on the levator hiatus seen on the axial plane (**b**)

facilities associated with the technique. Thereafter, within the same session (or within the subsequent week) for better diagnostic confidence, in less than 30 min the patient may undergo a complete check of her postdelivery pelvic anatomy by static MRI, including depiction of fat recesses, muscular attachments to the endopelvic fascia, perineal body position, paraurethral ligaments, and pudendal nerve course. Should occult changes be revealed, a rehabilitative program can be set up or planned, accordingly.

6.3.2 Second Step (Within 6 Months)

A double, anatomical, and functional MRI investigation is performed to compare pelvic structure anatomy at early postdelivery to that at post-recovery period and to detect any functional disorder affecting voiding and/or evacuation (Fig. 6.7) and pelvic organs stability as well. Again, in case of abnormality, a tailored therapeutic planning can be adopted, including both conservative and minimally invasive surgical approach.

6.3.3 Third Step (Within the Subsequent Three Decades)

A timely spaced 2-D TPUS study (Fig. 6.8) is performed every 4–5 years, unless otherwise needed for unexpected complains, for both optimal follow-up of therapy and in order to prevent the need for more invasive surgical procedures.

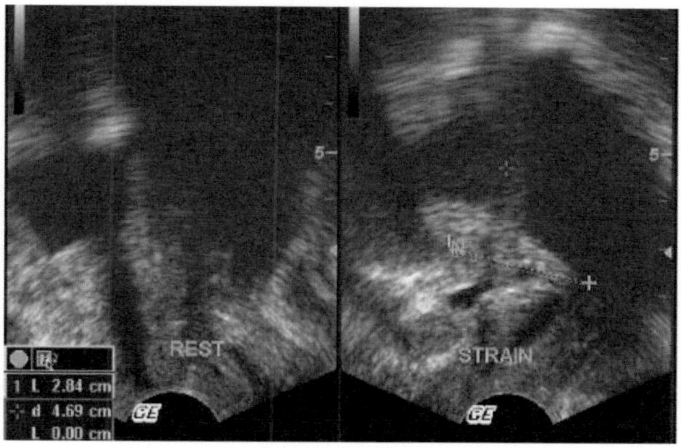

Fig. 6.8 Hypermobility (symphysis-to-neck distance >2.8 cm) of posterior bladder base and urethra on straining seen by routine 2D TPUS in a 58-year-old multiparous woman with occasional episodes of stress urinary incontinence of recent onset

Conclusions

Although the clinical assessment remains the first line investigation for the diagnosis of child birth trauma after vaginal delivery, diagnostic imaging tools, by either anal endosonography, 3-D TPUS or MRI, are more and more frequently considered today in order to help physicians to take adequate decision for therapy planning. Despite proper recognition and primary repair of acute obstetric anal sphincter injuries, up to 34–91 % women have been reported to exhibit persistent anal sphincter defects on ultrasound within 3 months of delivery. As such, given the high rate of occult changes in asymptomatic women after their first vaginal delivery and the awareness that the bulk of recovery takes place within the subsequent 6 months, a reasonable primary prevention strategy for the general female population is highly desirable. The common belief that routine imaging assessment of pelvic anatomy, either by 3-D TPUS or static and dynamic MRI, should be undertaken only in those with clinical concern of pelvic floor damage or in those who undergo prolapse surgery can no longer be sustained. At present, the following question arises: does the IFIP protocol described above influence women outcomes better after vaginal delivery and prove crucial in the future to prevent them from developing overt pelvic floor dysfunctions with advancing age? Hopefully, the required clinical studies will begin sooner.

References

1. Minini G, Zanelli S, Inselvini P et al (2010) Mechanism of pelvic floor trauma during vaginal delivery. In: Santoro GA, Wieczorek AP, Bartram CI (eds) Pelvic floor disorders, vol 12. Springer-Verlag Italia, Milan, pp 137–141
2. Kearney R, Miller JM, Ashton-Miller JA, DeLancey JOL (2006) Obstetric factors associated with levator ani muscle injury after vaginal birth. Obstet Gynecol 107:144–149
3. Lien K-C, Mooney B, DeLancey JOL, Ashton-Miller JA (2004) Levator ani muscle stretch induced by simulated vagina birth. Obstet Gynecol 103:31–40

4. Yousuf AA, DeLancey JOL, Brandon CJ et al (2009) Pelvic structure and function at 1 month compared to 7 months by dynamic magnetic resonance after vaginal birth. Am J Obstet Gynecol 201:514.e1–514.e7
5. Tunn R, DeLancey JOL, Howard D et al (1999) MR imaging of levator ani muscle recovery following vaginal delivery. Int Urogynecol J Pelvic Floor Dysfunct 10:300–307
6. Haylen BT, de Ridder D, Freeman RM et al (2009) An international urogynecological association (IUGA)/international continence society (ICS) joint report on the terminology for female pelvic floor dysfunction. Neurourol Urodyn 29:4–20
7. Stark M, Bohe M, Valentin L (2003) Results of endosonographic imaging of the anal sphincter 2–7 days after primary repair of third- or fourth-degree obstetric sphincter tears. Ultrasound Obstet Gynecol 22:609–615
8. Stark M, Bohe M, Fortling B et al (2005) Endosonography of the anal sphincter in women of different age and parity. Ultrasound Obstet Gynecol 25:169–176
9. Christensen AF, Nyhuus B, Nielsen MB et al (2005) Three-dimensional anal endosonography may improve diagnostic confidence of detecting damage to the anal sphincter complex. Br J Radiol 78:308–311
10. Faltin DL, Boulvain M, Irion O et al (2000) Diagnosis of anal sphincter tears by postpartum endosonography to predict fecal incontinence. Obstet Gynecol 95:643–647
11. Sultan AH, Thakar R (2007) Third and fourth degree tears. In: Sultan AH, Thakar R, Fenner D (eds) Perineal and anal sphincter trauma. Springer, London, pp 33–51
12. Dietz HP, Steensma AB, Hastings R (2003) Three-dimensional ultrasound imaging of the pelvic floor: the effect of parturition on paravaginal support structures. Ultrasound Obstet Gynecol 21:589–595
13. Dietz H (2007) Quantification of major morphological abnormalities of the levator ani. Ultrasound Obstet Gynecol 29:329–334
14. DeLancey JOL, Kearney R, Chou Q et al (2003) The appearance of levator ani muscle abnormalities in magnetic resonance images after vaginal delivery. Obstet Gynecol 101:46–53
15. DeLancey JOL (1999) Structural anatomy of the posterior pelvic compartment as it relates to rectocele. Am J Obstet Gynecol 180:815–823
16. Dietz H, Shek K, Clarke B (2005) Biometry of the pubovisceral muscle and levator hiatus by three-dimensional pelvic floor ultrasound. Ultrasound Obstet Gynecol 25:580–585
17. Lienemann A, Anthuber C, Baron A et al (1997) Dynamic MR colpocystorectography assessing pelvic-floor descent. Eur Radiol 7:1309–1317
18. Huddleston HT, Dunnihoo DR, Huddleston PM et al (1995) Magnetic resonance imaging of defects in DeLancey's vaginal support levels I, II and II. Am J Obstet Gynecol 172:1778–1784
19. Kim JK, Kim YJ, Choo MS et al (2003) The urethra and its supporting structures in women with stress urinary incontinence: MR imaging using an endovaginal coil. AJR Am J Roentgenol 180:1037–1044
20. Piloni V, Bergamasco M, Bregolin F et al (2014) MR imaging of the pudendal nerve: a one-year experience on an outpatient basis. Pelviperineology 33:54–59
21. Hsu Y, Summers A, Hussain HK et al (2006) Levator plate angle in women with pelvic organ prolapse compared to women with normal support using dynamic MR imaging. Am J Obstet Gynecol 194:1427–1433
22. Bump RC, Mattiasson A, Bo K et al (1996) The standardization of terminology of female pelvic organ prolapse and pelvic floor dysfunction. Am J Obstet Gynecol 175:10–17
23. Comiter GV, Vasavada SP, Barbaric ZL et al (1999) Grading pelvic prolapse and pelvic floor relaxation using dynamic magnetic resonance imaging. Urology 54:454–457
24. Singh K, Reid WMN, Berger LA (2001) Assessment and grading of pelvic organ prolapse by use of dynamic resonance imaging. Am J Obstet Gynecol 185:71–77
25. DeLancey JOL, Hurd WW (1998) Size of the urogenital hiatus in the levator ani muscles in normal women and women with pelvic organ prolapse. Obstet Gynecol 91:364–368
26. Pannu HP, Kaufman HS, Cundiff GW et al (2000) Dynamic MR imaging of pelvic organ prolapse: spectrum of abnormalities. Radiographics 20:1567–1582

7 Pelvic Floor EMG: Principles, Techniques, and Applications

Roberto Merletti

7.1 Introduction

The anal sphincter and the puborectalis are the most important muscles providing fecal continence. The anal sphincter comprises an internal involuntary smooth muscle layer (IAS) and an external voluntary striated muscle layer (EAS).

Obstetric lesions are often associated to sphincter tears, that is spontaneous or iatrogenous direct lesions of the muscle tissue. However, other lesions, less investigated and discussed in the literature, may involve the innervation of the EAS, rather than the muscle itself, and may be caused by tissue stretching or cutting (episiotomy). They often result in muscle denervation which may (or may not) be followed by a variable degree of reinnervation and often lead to loss of muscle control by the CNS, a situation functionally similar to a muscle tear. Since the axons innervating the EAS are too small to be seen, the damage cannot be prevented, detected or documented without recently developed instrumentation. Such an instrumentation is based on the automatic detection of the innervation zones (IZ) of the motor units of the EAS. A motor unit comprises a motor neuron and the muscle fibers it innervates. The ensemble of the neuromuscular junctions (NMJ) between the axonal branches and the muscle fibers of a motor unit is called the IZ of that motor unit.

It is not known how many motor units exist in the EAS but it is known that they are arranged circularly and they are innervated either at one end or somewhere along their length. The European Project "On Asimmetry of Sphincters (OASIS)" demonstrated, in 2005, that there is a large inter-individual variability of motor unit and IZ arrangement among subjects of both genders [1, 2]. The innervation pattern of the puborectalis was investigated within the same project [3].

R. Merletti
Department of Electronics and Telecommunications, Laboratory for Engineering of the Neuromuscular System (LISiN), Politecnico di Torino, Torin, Italy
e-mail: roberto.merletti@polito.it

D. Riva, G. Minini (eds.), *Childbirth-Related Pelvic Floor Dysfunction: Risk Factors, Prevention, Evaluation, and Treatment*,
DOI 10.1007/978-3-319-18197-4_7

Episiotomy may cut some of the axons or axonal branches innervating the EAS and cause weakening of the muscle, possibly resulting in incontinence at a later age. It is therefore important to know where the IZs are located in order to plan in advance if mediolateral episiotomy should be performed and, if so, whether the right or left side should be preferred. The same technology could of course be used to document the course or reinnervation and the residual damage. Knowledge of the innervation pattern of the puborectalis muscle, not involved in episiotomy, may be of interest in colo-rectal surgery.

The technology for the identification of the IZs of a muscle is based on electrophysiological considerations that will be described in Sect. 7.2 of this chapter. The remaining sessions will primarily describe the state of the art and the applications of a novel electrophysiological technology to the prevention of child-deliver-related lesions and incontinence. This application has been the topic of the project "Technologies for anal sphincter analysis and incontinence (TASI)" [4, 5].

7.2 Basic Electrophysiological Concepts Concerning Fusiform and Circular Muscles

7.2.1 Intra-muscular and Noninvasive Detection Techniques

The EAS muscle, as most other muscles, has been investigated with the traditional coaxial needle technique [6, 7]. A few needle insertions are required to collect representative information from the muscle. This technique provides information about individual motor units and has a very small detection volume (about 1 mm^3). It does not provide information about the location of motor unit IZs. Minimally invasive detection systems based on intra-anal probes have been developed more than 10 years ago [1, 2, 8, 9] within the framework of the European Project "On Asymmetry in Sphincters (OASIS)". These systems provide a greater detection volume as well as information about motor unit geometry and IZ. The technique is based on the detection of propagating action potentials along the fibers of the motor units of muscles; technical details are provided in a number of publications [1, 2, 4, 5, 8, 9] as well as in textbooks [10, 11].

This noninvasive technique and its application will be shortly reviewed in the following subsection.

7.2.2 Single Fiber and Motor Unit Action Potentials in Muscles with Fibers Parallel to the Detection Array

A muscle fiber has a membrane resting potential of about −70 mV (internal negative). When the action potential of a neuron reaches the terminal branches of the axon and each neuromuscular junction, the release of acetylcholine locally leads to inversion of the membrane polarity and triggers an action potential into each of the innervated muscle fibers. Figure 7.1a describes the local generation of an action potential along a muscle fiber. This region of membrane depolarization widens

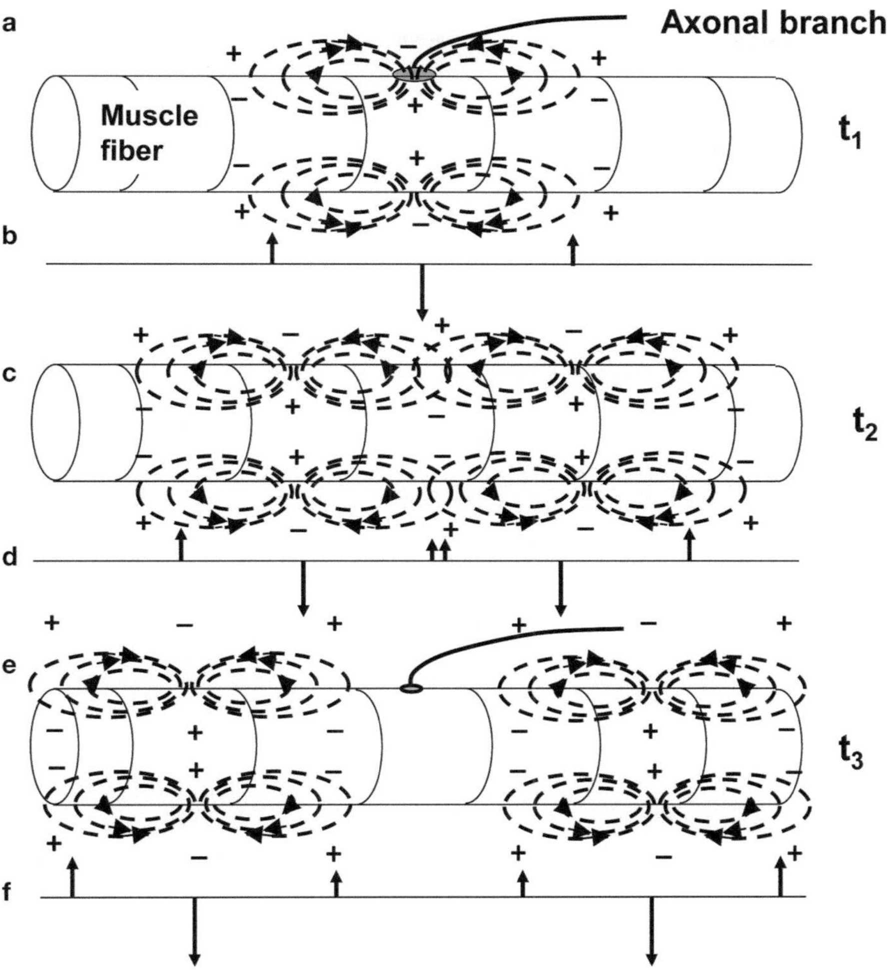

Fig. 7.1 Generation and propagation of an action potential (AP) in a cylindrical muscle fiber. (**a**) The axonal branch releases acetylcholine at the neuromuscular junction (NMJ), and triggers the AP. The underlying membrane depolarizes generating current loops that extend the depolarization to nearby regions of the cell. (**b**) The current "poles" corresponding to this situation at time t_1 are depicted. *Upward arrows* indicate currents exiting the muscle fiber and depolarizing the membrane, *downward arrows* indicate currents entering the muscle fiber and repolarizing the membrane. (**c**) Two APs are being generated in space and propagate in opposite directions as the NMJ area repolarizes (time t_2). (**d**) The current "poles" corresponding to the situation at time t_2 are depicted: two tripoles are generated. (**e**) The two APs are fully generated and travel in opposite directions towards the tendon junctions. (**f**) Two separate current tripoles describe the propagating APs at time t_3 (Reproduced with permission from Fig. 3.4 of [10])

while its center repolarizes, therefore generating two depolarized regions propagating toward the ends of the fiber, as indicated in Fig. 7.1c, e where the dashed lines represent current flows. The arrows in Fig. 7.1b, d, f indicate current inflows and outflows across the muscle cell membrane. As a first approximation, a

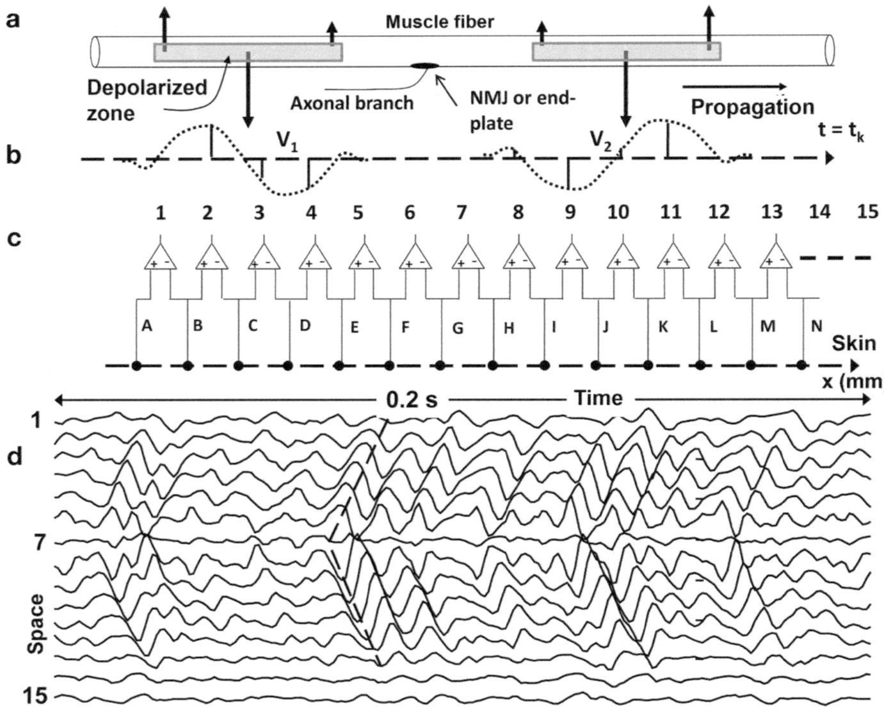

Fig. 7.2 Generation of multichannel EMG. (**a**) Single muscle fiber with two depolarized zones (current tripoles) propagating in opposite directions starting from the neuromuscular junction (see Fig. 7.1e, f). (**b**) Analog differential voltage detected on the skin, due to the propagating tripoles, and instantaneous samples in space provided by the amplifier array at a fixed time instant $t=t_k$. (**c**) Array of differential amplifiers connected to an array of electrodes placed on the skin (A-N). Note that signals propagating in the right direction see the non-inverting input first and then the inverting input while the opposite happens for signals propagating in the left direction. (**d**) Set of real EMG signals acquired with a linear electrode array (such as the A-N array) from the biceps brachii muscle. The 1-15 channels correspond to the 1-15 output signals of the differential amplifiers versus time. Many propagating potentials, generated by many motor units, can be identified. It is interesting to observe that all the motor units are innervated under channel 7 and extend over the entire muscle length. Channels 14 and 15 are over the distal tendon area. The *dashed lines* represent the "signature" of a motor unit. Inter-electrode distance = 10 mm

propagating depolarized zone can be represented by a current tripole whose poles add up to zero net current.

Let us now consider two depolarized regions (two current tripoles) moving along a muscle fiber parallel to the skin as indicated in Fig. 7.2a. The two potential distributions resulting on the skin, due to these sources, are depicted in Fig. 7.2b.

Consider the array of electrodes A-N and differential amplifiers with outputs 1-15 depicted in Fig. 7.2c. The propagating action potential generated by one fiber and detected by this set of differential amplifiers, at a given time instant, is depicted in Fig. 7.2b. The fibers innervated by branches of the same axon, forming a motor unit, generate a motor unit action potential (MUAP) which is the sum of the single fiber action potentials associated to each discharge of the neuron. Figure 7.2d shows

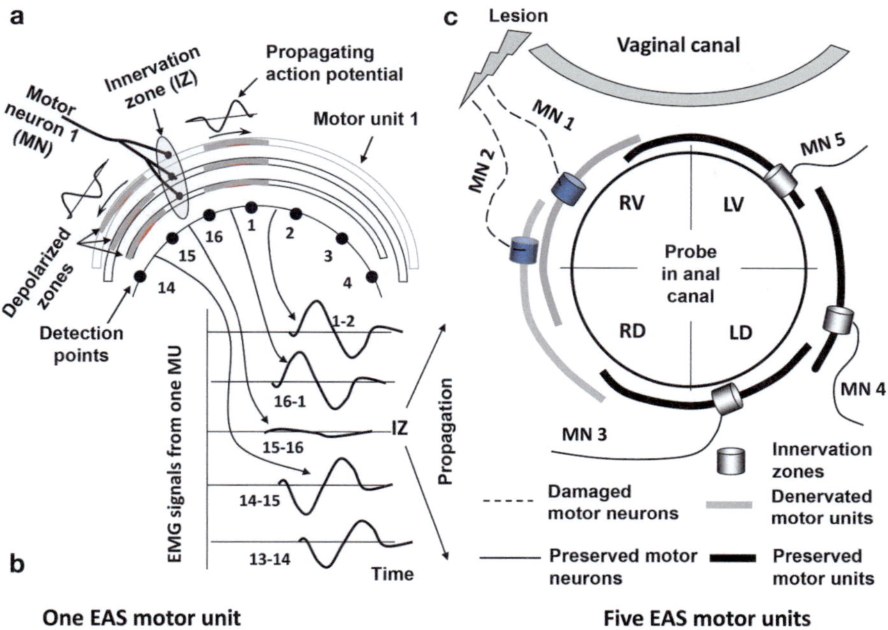

Fig. 7.3 Schematic diagram of the arrangements of motor units of the external anal sphincter (EAS). (**a**) One motor unit (motorneuron 1 and muscle fibers). (**b**) Differential signals detected by electrode pairs placed on the circumference of a cylindrical probe inserted in the anal canal (see Fig. 7.4). (**c**) Schematic diagram of the arrangements of five motor units of the EAS. Two of these motor units are innervated by motor neurons (*MN1 and MN2*) comprised in the right-ventral quadrant (*RV*) of the EAS, two are innervated by motor neurons (*MN3 and MN4*) comprised in the left dorsal quadrant (*LD*) of the EAS and one by a motor neuron (*MN5*) in the left ventral quadrant of the EAS. A right mediolateral episiotomy would likely damage or interrupt MN1 and MN2 and denervate the corresponding motor units. A left right mediolateral episiotomy would likely damage or interrupt MN5

a 0.2 s segment of multichannel EMG detected by the array of Fig. 7.2c placed on a biceps brachii muscle. An example of MUAP is identified by dashed lines in Fig. 7.2d, together with many other MUAPs generated by motor units of the same muscle with fibers parallel to the skin. All motor units are innervated under channel 7 and terminate beyond channel 1 and at channel 13. Channels 14 and 15 are above one of the tendons. The other tendon is beyond channel 1. Figure 7.2d provides a space-time (y versus t) representation of "firings" of many motor units (MUAPs) as detected by an electrode array placed on the skin along the muscle fiber direction. Each trace represents the signal detected by one electrode pair (1-15).

In the case of the anal sphincter muscle the motor units are arranged in a circular pattern and so are the electrodes, as depicted in Figs. 7.3 and 7.4. Figure 7.3a shows a motor unit spanning channels 14 to 4 of a circular electrode array. The IZ is "under" electrodes 15-16 and propagation is detected up to past electrodes 14 (counterclockwise) and 4 (clockwise). Five motor units are schematically depicted in Fig. 7.3c, each with different length and innervation zone location. If motoneurons MN1 and MN2 are cut by the episiotomy surgery ("lesion" in Fig. 7.3c) the

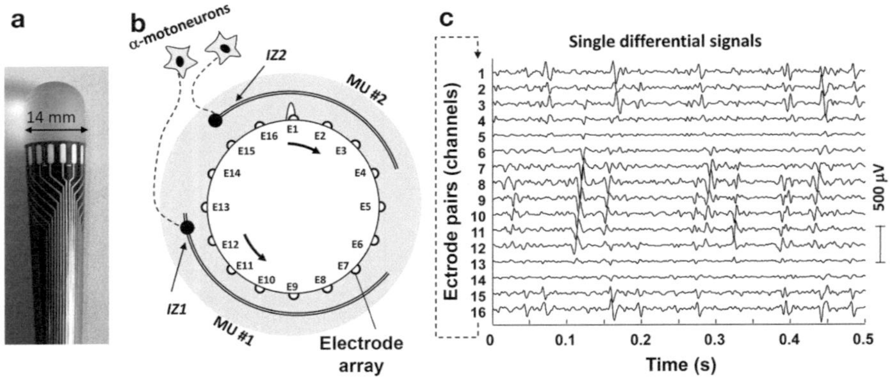

Fig. 7.4 (**a**) Intra-anal probe with 16 circumferential electrodes. (**b**) Cross-sectional view of the electrode array and schematic representation of two motor units. (**c**) Example of anal sphincter EMG differential signals. Two motor units can be identified (among others): the first is innervated at one end under channel 13 and extends to channel 6, the second is innervated at one end under channel 15 and extends to channel 4. Other motor units can be identified and their innervation zone can be localized (Permission from [9], Fig. 1, page 114)

corresponding motor units are denervated and may or may not be re-innervated after surgery. A commercially available EAS probe is depicted in Fig. 7.4a and an example of experimental signals is depicted in Fig. 7.4c. It is evident, from Fig. 7.4c, that in this EAS muscle there are two main IZs: one under channel 14-15 with clockwise propagation and one under channel 12-13 with counterclockwise propagation (channel 1 is anterior and channel 9 is posterior).

It has been shown that the innervation of the EAS sphincter is very variable from subject to subject [1, 4, 5, 9]. Examples of schematic and real propagating MUAPs are provided in Fig. 7.5.

Figure 7.5a schematically depicts the MUAP pattern of motor units innervated under channel 5 and under channel 12-13 while Fig. 7.5b shows a case of innervation under channel 8 and a case of innervation under channel 1-16. Figure 7.5c depicts a set of experimental signals showing a number of MUs innervated under channels 2, 12, 1-3, 1-16. Figure 7.6 shows a circular histogram of the distribution of IZs of 2,748 motor units observed in 500 pregnant women [4, 5] indicating that the ventral side of the EAS is the least innervated while the right and left hemisphincters have rich innervation which is highly variable from person to person [1].

7.3 Results of Recent Studies on the Innervation of the External Anal Sphincter and Puborectalis Muscles

Since the distribution of IZs of the EAS shows a very high inter-subject variability [1] no general rule can be proposed in favor of right or left or midline episiotomy. Figure 7.7 depicts four examples of EAS innervation and related episiotomy risks. Figure 7.7a depicts a case of bilateral hemisphincter innervation implying a

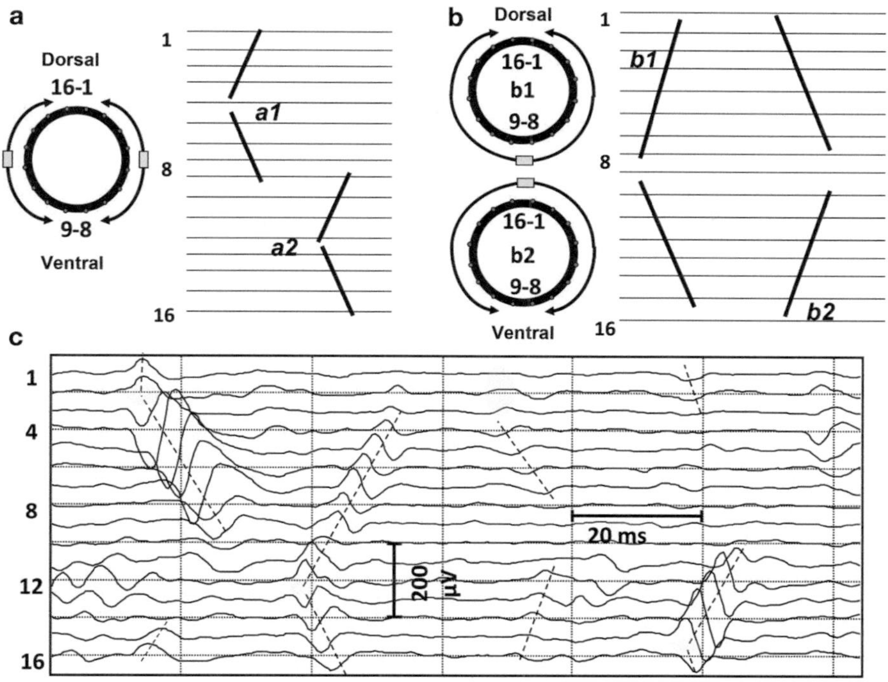

Fig. 7.5 (**a**) Schematic representation of innervation zones and propagation directions of two motor units, one in the right and one in the left hemisphincter. (**b**) Schematic representation of innervation zones and propagation directions of two long motor units, one innervated under channel 8 and one innervated under channel 1-16. (**c**) Experimental signals showing motor units innervated under channel 2-3, under channel 12, under channel 1-3 and under channel 15. Consider that, due to the circular probe, channel 1 is next to channel 16

medium risk for a short incision, Fig. 7.7b depicts a case of high risk due to innervation being concentrated in the rectovaginal septum (perineum), Fig. 7.7c depicts a case of dorsal innervation of the EAS and therefore low risk, while Fig. 7.7d depicts a case of innervation in the left-ventral quadrant implying a high risk of a left mediolateral episiotomy and a much lower risk of a right mediolateral episiotomy; of course the opposite holds for a single innervation region in the right-ventral quadrant of the EAS.

The technique described in [12–14] and summarized in Sect. 7.2.2 of this chapter, was adopted in the double blind study ("Technologies for anal sphincter analysis and incontinence (TASI)") [5] carried out on 331 pregnant women, 86 of which underwent mediolateral episiotomy (82 on the right side, 4 on the left side). One of these cases is outlined in Fig. 7.8. Figure 7.8a shows the arrangement of nine motor units and of their IZs, identified as described in Sect. 7.2.2, 6 weeks before delivery and 6 weeks after delivery. For methodological details see [14]. Despite the evidence of major denervation and of EAS EMG asymmetry, this woman was not incontinent at the time of the second evaluation.

Fig. 7.6 Circular histogram of the location of innervation zones of 2748 motor units identified in the external anal sphincter of 500 women. The distribution is bimodal with higher likelihood of innervation zones in the right and left hemisphincter (Reproduced with permission from [4])

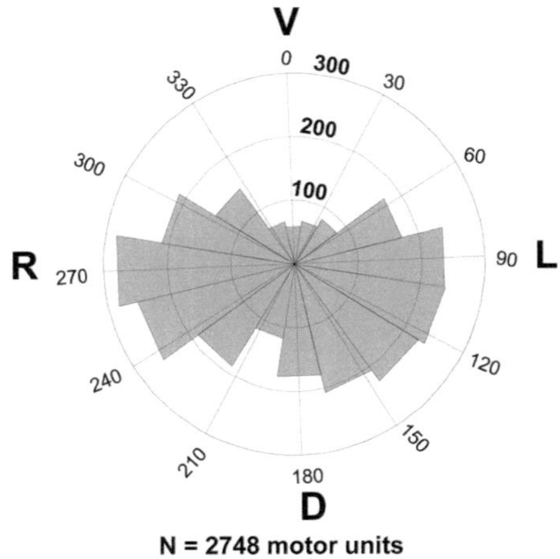

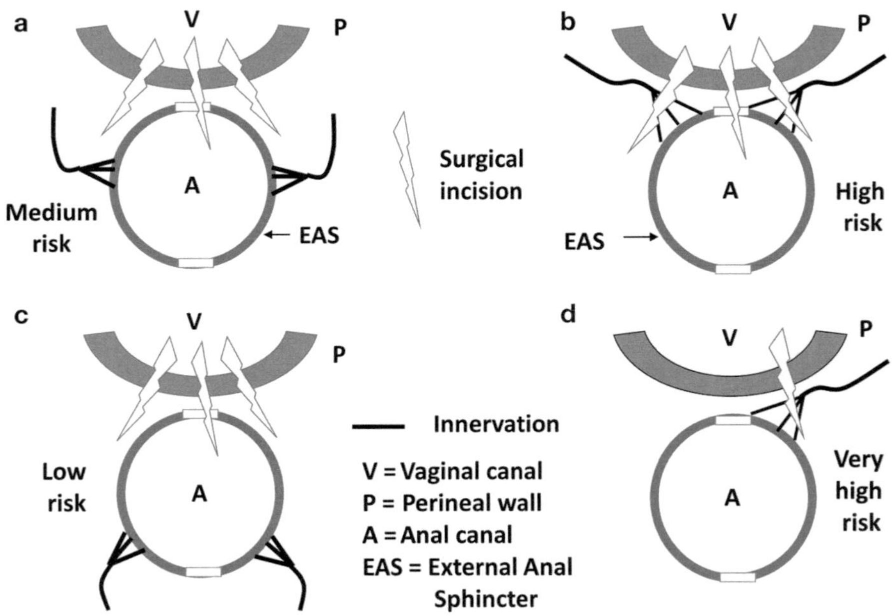

Fig. 7.7 Four innervation modalities of the anal sphincter with four different risks levels related to episiotomy. (**a**) Innervation zones concentrated in the right and left hemisphincter: risk is moderate and depends on the pattern of the axonal branches. (**b**) Innervation zones in the right and left ventral quadrants of the sphincter: the risk of partial denervation of the sphincter due to episiotomy is high, regardless of the side. (**c**) Innervation zones in the right and left dorsal quadrants of the sphincter: the risk of partial denervation of the sphincter due to episiotomy is low, regardless of the side. (**d**) Innervation zones in the left ventral quadrant of the sphincter: the risk of denervation of the sphincter is high if a left mediolateral episiotomy is performed and low if a right mediolateral episiotomy is performed. A mirror-like situation implies high risk of denervation if a right mediolateral episiotomy is performed reprinted with permission from Di Vella G, Riva D, Merletti R. Incontinenza dello sfintere anale sterno da episiotomia e prevenzione del danno iatrogeno. Riv It Med Leg. 2015; 37(2):473–489

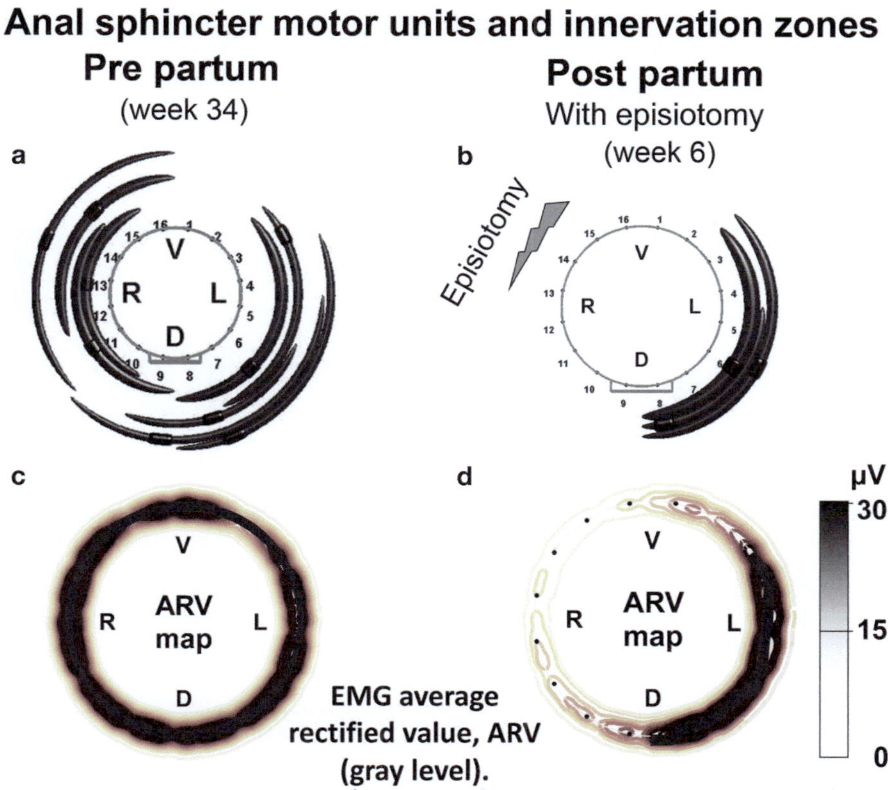

Fig. 7.8 (**a**, **b**) Distribution of nine motor units and of their innervation zones before and after delivery with right mediolateral episiotomy. (**c**, **d**) The thickness of the *black arcs* indicate the average rectified value of the EMG. Despite the major denervation the woman was not incontinent 6 weeks after delivery (Reproduced from [5])

Depending on the individual EAS innervation pattern, episiotomy may or may not imply alterations of such pattern. In some cases, random factors, posture or different contraction modalities might even cause the involvement of a greater number of motor units in the postpartum condition. Statistical considerations are therefore required. Figure 7.9a shows the prepartum distribution of IZs of 82 women who underwent episiotomy. The postpartum distribution of IZ is depicted in Fig. 7.9b. The decrement on the number of IZ in the RV quadrant of the EAS is evident and statistically significant ($p < 0.05$) whereas it is not in the other quadrants (see also Fig. 7.10b and [5] for issues related to EAS tears). Figure 7.10 compares the changes between pre- postpartum number of IZs in each EAS quadrant in the case of cesarean delivery (60 cases) and episiotomy (82 cases). No significant changes are observed in the first case while a statistically significant change is observed in the RV quadrant of the EAS in the second case. Nevertheless, cesarean delivery is not necessarily preventive of EAs damage [15].

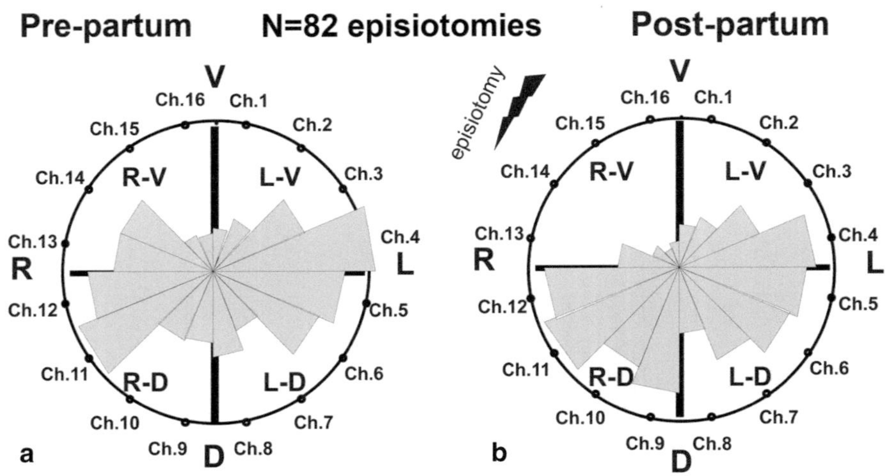

Fig. 7.9 Circular histogram of the distribution of innervation zones in the anal sphincter of 82 women before and after child delivery with right mediolateral episiotomy. A reduction of innervation zones in the right-ventral (*RV*) quadrant of the sphincter is evident and is statistically significant (see Fig. 7.10b) while changes in other quadrants are not reprinted with permission from Di Vella G, Riva D, Merletti R. Incontinenza dello sfintere anale sterno da episiotomia e prevenzione del danno iatrogeno. Riv It Med Leg. 2015; 37(2):473–489

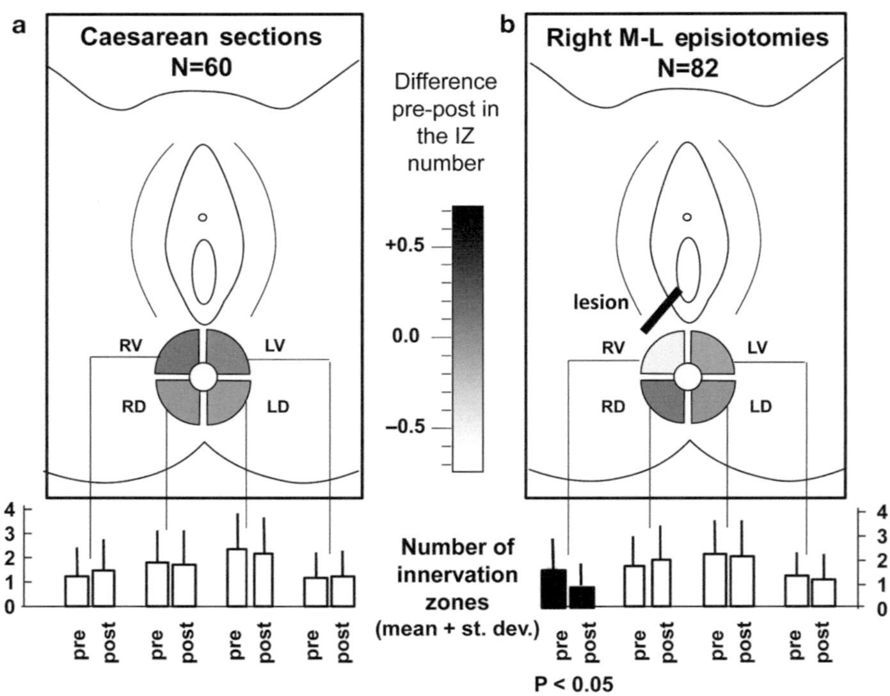

Fig. 7.10 Mean and standard deviation of the number of motor units identified with innervations in each of the four quadrants of the anal sphincter. (**a**) Pre- and postpartum with cesarean delivery (60 subjects). (**b**) Pre- and postpartum with right mediolateral episiotomy (82 subjects). The only pre--post difference that is statistically significant concerns the number of IZ in the right-ventral (*RV*) quadrant in the episiotomy cases (Reproduced from [5])

The puborectalis muscle is the second most important muscle providing continence. This muscle is not affected by episiotomy but may be stretched by pregnancy. It might easily be investigated, with the same minimally invasive technique, with an electrode array applied on a gloved finger [3].

7.4 The Controversial Issue of Episiotomy: Analysis of the Literature

Episiotomy is a controversial practice which is applied routinely in some countries (Latin America and Eastern Europe) and more rarely in others (Scandinavian Countries) with the purpose of reducing the stress of the newborn and the likelihood of perineal and sphincter tears which are difficult to suture. Right mediolateral episiotomy is by far more common than left mediolateral episiotomy because it is more easily performed by a right-handed person. Mediolateral episiotomies angled closer to the midline are significantly associated with anal sphincter injuries (26° vs. 37°, $p=0.01$) [17, 18]. Standard obstetric and midwifery texts indicate that a mediolateral episiotomy should be at least 40° from the midline but doctors and midwifes follow different rules [16]. If episiotomy is performed at the proper angle (45° to 60° from the midline) [16–18] it is unlikely that the EAS is directly damaged, nevertheless the axons and their terminal branches innervating the muscle may be cut, resulting in more or less extensive EAS denervation which may or may not be followed by reinnervation in the first few weeks after delivery [34]. This damage may lead to increased likelihood of fecal incontinence (FI) in later years [19].

Women with anal sphincter tears are more than twice as likely to report postpartum fecal incontinence than women without sphincter tears [20]. Anal sphincter tears occur in 2–19 % of vaginal deliveries [21], however limited information is available on episiotomy-related EAS denervation which may have similar consequences on voluntary muscle control.

Several studies have demonstrated that midline episiotomy is an independent risk factor for sphincter injuries [22]. Mediolateral episiotomy is controversial, since some studies showed it to be an independent risk factor [23, 24] whereas others found it to be protective for fecal incontinence in primiparous women [25]. Very likely the lack of consensus is related to two factors: (a) that no midwife and only 22 % of the doctors perform truly mediolateral episiotomies [26] and (b) the angle may influence the direct damage to the muscle but is not correlated to innervation damage.

The works of Enck, Franz and Wietek [1, 2, 27, 28] suggest that either natural or iatrogenic asymmetry of innervation of the EAS contributes to the occurrence and severity of incontinence symptoms resulting from aging or pelvic floor trauma, after child delivery.

The association of pelvic floor trauma to child delivery modality (in particular to episiotomy), is discussed in many studies [20, 22, 25, 29–32]. The concept is that stretching or laceration or cutting of the nerve twigs may lead to the same consequences of stretching, laceration and cutting of muscle tissue and either or both may be present. Furthermore, surgical muscle repair does not imply functional recovery if muscle denervation is present.

Although EAS denervation consequent to mediolateral episiotomy can now be ascertained [5], its role in determining FI at a later age is still being investigated [21, 32–43]. Despite this extensive literature, no indication is provided about the criterion that should be used regarding which side should episiotomy be performed on. Thus, episiotomy is usually performed on the right side. Knowledge of the side to be preferred (if any), based on the electrophysiological test described above might reduce the consequences of this intervention and possibly increase the consensus about the procedure [5].

The literature quoted above focuses on minimization of direct potential damage to the EAS muscle and does not consider its innervation modality. Data reported in Figs. 7.8 and 7.9 suggest that tear and denervation may result in similar functional effects since both disable a portion of the EAS.

In conclusion, prepartum screening of the EAS innervation and the recording of this information on a "perineal card," could "guide" episiotomy (when strictly required) and likely reduce the prevalence of FI in women at a later age and the disagreement about its origin.

7.5 Epidemiological and Economic Aspects, Technology Transfer, and Dissemination

As reported by T. Wheeler et al. in their excellent review [24] , the prevalence of FI in community-dwelling adult women is 0.4–18 % [44], with an estimated direct cost of diagnosis and treatment of US$17,000 per patient [45].

Bharucha et al. [54] did a survey on 2,800 white US women and found that 1 in 15 had moderate to severe FI but only 48 % had consulted a physician in the previous year. The prevalence increased with age from 7 % (third decade of life) to 22 % (sixth decade of life) and was stable thereafter. The problem may be more frequent than is commonly believed, with an economic and social cost greater than it appears.

According to Weber et al. [55] FI affects between 1 and 16 % of women, with prevalence increasing with age. The most common cause of FI in otherwise healthy women is damage to the anal sphincter during childbirth. Prevention of FI should be the first research priority for gynecologists. Routine midline (median) episiotomy has no place in modern obstetrics; when episiotomy must be performed for obstetric indications, use of mediolateral episiotomy should result in fewer anal sphincter injuries than use of midline episiotomy. A general research priority is to understand the independent factors in FI so as to identify modifiable risk factors in women.

Evidence regarding the use of mediolateral episiotomy has not been established in preventing sphincter tears and therefore social and economic costs. A 1999 Cochrane Review, which used severe perineal trauma as an outcome, failed to find differences between restrictive versus midline or mediolateral episiotomies [29]. According to a JAMA review [46], no evidence supports episiotomy as preventive practice to avoid pelvic floor damage. In two cohort studies women were asked about anal incontinence [23, 47]. Neither study found episiotomy to be statistically associated with reduced risk of incontinence of stool or flatus; rather, an aggregate of the two studies suggests an almost twofold increase in risk (mean odds ratio: 1.91; 95 % CI: 1.03–3.56) [46].

According to Signorello et al. [19], women who had episiotomy had a higher risk of FI at 3 (mean odds ratio: 5.5, 95 % CI: 1.8–16.2) and 6 (mean odds ratio: 3.7, 95 % CI: 0.9–15.6) months postpartum compared with women with an intact perineum. Compared with women with a spontaneous laceration, episiotomy tripled the risk of FI at 3 months and 6 months postpartum. These authors concluded that midline episiotomy is not effective in protecting the perineum and sphincters during childbirth, and may impair anal continence. The estimates of prevalence of postpartum FI range from 3 % to 42 % [48–59].

In 2005 Deutekom et al. [51] estimated the average cost of an incontinent person at about 2,169 euro/year including personal and societal costs. In 2007 Sung et al. [52] estimated this cost as near 6,000 US$/year and per patient for a total health cost of 57,500,000 US $/year.

Because of the insufficiency and variability of the available economic data it is impossible, at the moment, to estimate the possible savings resulting from a policy of no episiotomy [53], a policy of planned minimal-risk episiotomy using an electrophysiological test [5] and a policy of routine episiotomy, but it seems that the second option is promising also from the point of view of economic and social cost.

Like most interdisciplinary technologies, the minimally invasive method to estimate EAS innervation, and consequently plan the least risky episiotomy modality long before child delivery (in case it will be deemed necessary), is not easily accepted by busy clinicians and obstetricians. Although the test is simple, fast and inexpensive, some ability to read and double-check the signals and the information displayed by the instrumentation is required (as is for the interpretation of ECG or EEG or evoked potentials). Despite the 10-year research experience and many publications, teaching of the technique is still limited. This fact results in a very limited demand, lack of a market and absence of interest by companies manufacturing medical equipment. In turn this results in no commercial pressure and no teaching. It is hoped that insurance companies, clinical and scientific associations, academic institutions and maternity centers would soon become aware of the large body of scientific literature concerning episiotomy and the proper way of performing it. A greater awareness of the problem by the gynecologists and obstetricians, especially in the countries where episiotomy is almost routinely applied, would certainly avoid legal issues dealing with the consequences of this controversial intervention. Information of medical students and clinical specialists and their training in properly performing prepartum tests and episiotomy is highly desirable.

Conclusions

Minimally invasive EMG of the EAS is a sufficiently tested technique to minimize episiotomy risks and document changes in EAS innervation/reinnervation patterns following obstetric trauma.

Its application should be extended to provide a prognosis for functional recovery following surgical repair of sphincter tears which is not useful in case of a denervated muscle. Dissemination of the method, teaching and training of operators are justified by recent findings. Potential reduction of cases of incontinence and economic and social costs, although not yet documented, should be expected.

Acknowledgments The author is grateful to Prof Taian Vieira, and to the partners of Project TASI [4, 5] for contributing material and data. The clinical advice and revision by Dr D. Riva are greatly appreciated. This chapter is extensively based on material published in Chap. 14 "Applications in proctology and obstetrics" of the book "Surface electromyography: physiology, engineering and applications" R. Merletti and D Farina editors, J Wiley and IEEE press 2015 and on material published in the book "Atlas of muscle innervation zones: understanding surface electromyography and its applications" by M. Barbero, R. Merletti and A. Rainoldi, published by Springer Verlag (2012). The author is grateful to Springer Verlag, John Wiley and IEEE Press for permission to reproduce material from these books. Project TASI as well as the preparation of this chapter were financially supported by Compagnia di San Paolo, Torino, Italy.

References

1. Enck P, Franz H, Azpiroz F, Fernandez-Fraga X, Hinninghofen H, Kaske-Bretag K, Bottin A, Martina S, Merletti R (2004) Innervation zones of the external anal sphincter in healthy male and female subjects. Digestion 69:123–130
2. Enck P, Hinninghofen H, Wietek H, Becker HD (2004) Functional asymmetry of pelvic floor innervation and its role in the pathogenesis of fecal incontinence. Digestion 69:102–111
3. Cescon C, Bottin A, Azpiroz F, Merletti R (2008) Detection of individual motor units of the puborectalis muscle by non-invasive EMG electrode arrays. J Electromyogr Kinesiol 28(3):382–389
4. Cescon C, Raimondi EE, Začesta V, Drusany-Starič K, Martsidis K, Merletti R (2014) Characterization of the motor units of the external anal sphincter in pregnant women with multichannel surface EMG. Int Urogynecol J 25:1097–1103
5. Cescon C, Riva D, Začesta V, Drusany-Starič K, Martsidis K, Protsepko O, Baessler K, Merletti R (2014) Effect of vaginal delivery on external anal sphincter muscle innervation pattern evaluated with multichannel surface EMG (results of the multicenter study TASI-2). Int Urogynecol J 25:1491–1499
6. López A, Nilsson BY, Mellgren A, Zetterström J, Holmström B (1999) Electromyography of the external anal sphincter: comparison between needle and surface electrodes. Dis Colon Rectum 42:482–485
7. Podnar S, Lukanovič A, Vodusek DB (2000) Anal sphincter electromyography after vaginal delivery: neuropathic insufficiency or normal wear and tear? Neurourol Urodyn 19:249–257
8. Enck P, Hinninghofen H, Merletti R, Azpiroz F (2005) The external anal sphincter and the role of surface electromyography. Neurogastroenterol Motil 17(Suppl 1):60–67
9. Merletti R, Bottin A, Cescon C, Farina D, Mesin L, Gazzoni M, Martina S, Pozzo M, Rainoldi A, Enck P (2004) Multichannel surface EMG for the non-invasive assessment of the anal sphincter muscle. Digestion 69:112–122
10. Barbero M, Merletti R, Rainoldi A (2012) Atlas of muscle innervation zones: understanding surface electromyography and its applications. Springer Verlag Italia. ISBN 978-88-470-2462-5
11. Merletti R, Farina D (eds.) (2015) Surface electromyography: physiology, engineering and applications. J Wiley and IEEE Press, NJ, USA
12. Cescon C, Mesin L, Nowakowski M, Merletti R (2011) Geometry assessment of anal sphincter muscle based on monopolar multichannel surface EMG signals. J Electromyogr Kinesiol 21(2):394–401

13. Enck P, Franz H, Davico E, Mastrangelo F, Mesin L, Merletti R (2010) Repeatability of innervation zone identification in the external anal sphincter muscle. Neurourol Urodyn 29(3): 449–457
14. Ullah K, Cescon C, Afsharipour B, Merletti R (2014) Automatic detection of motor unit innervation zones of the external anal sphincter by multichannel surface EMG. J Electromyogr Kinesiol 24(6):860–867
15. Nygaard I (2005) Should women be offered elective cesarean section in the hope of preserving pelvic floor function? Int Urogynecol J 16:253–254
16. Tincello D, Williams A, Fowler G, Adams E, Richmond D, Alfirevic Z (2003) Differences in episiotomy technique between midwives and doctors. BJOG 110(12):1041–1044
17. Kalis V, Karbanova J, Horak M, Lobovsky L, Kralickova M, Rokyta Z (2008) The incision angle of mediolateral episiotomy before delivery and after repair. Int J Gynaecol Obstet 103:5–8
18. Freeman RM, Hollands HJ, Barron L, Kapoor DS (2014) Cutting a mediolateral episiotomy at the correct angle: evaluation of a new device, the Episcissors-60. Med Devices (Auckl) 7:23–28
19. Signorello LB, Harlow BL, Chekos AK, Repke JT (2000) Midline episiotomy and anal incontinence: retrospective cohort study. BMJ 320(7227):86–90
20. Borello-France D, Burgio KL, Richter HE, Zyczynski H, Fitzgerald MP, Whitehead W, Fine P, Nygaard I, Handa VL, Visco AG, Weber AM, Brown MB (2006) Fecal and urinary incontinence in primiparous women. Obstet Gynecol 108(4):863–872
21. Fenner D (2006) Anal incontinence: relationship to pregnancy, vaginal delivery, and cesarean section. Semin Perinatol 30(5):261–266
22. Andrews V, Sultan AH, Thakar R, Jones PW (2006) Risk factors for obstetric anal sphincter injury: a prospective study. Birth 33(2):117–1122
23. Sartore A, De Seta F, Maso G, Pregazzi R, Grimaldi E, Guaschino S (2004) The effects of mediolateral episiotomy on pelvic floor function after vaginal delivery. Obstet Gynecol 103: 669–673
24. Wheeler TL, Richter HE (2007) Delivery method, anal sphincter tears and fecal incontinence: new information on a persistent problem. Curr Opin Obstet Gynecol 19(5):474–479
25. De Leeuw JW, Vierhout ME, Struijk PC, Hop WC, Wallenburg HC (2001) Anal sphincter damage after vaginal delivery: functional outcome and risk factors for fecal incontinence. Acta Obstet Gynecol Scand 80(9):830–834
26. Andrews V, Thakar R, Sultan A, Jones P (2005) Are mediolateral episiotomies actually mediolateral? BJOG 112:1156–1158
27. Franz H, Hinninghofen H, Kowalski A, Merletti R, Enck P (2006) Mode of delivery affects anal sphincter innervation. Gastroenterology 130(Suppl 2):S724
28. Wietek BM, Hinninghofen H, Jehle EC, Enck P, Franz HB (2007) Asymmetric sphincter innervation is associated with fecal incontinence after anal sphincter trauma during childbirth. Neurourol Urodyn 26(1):134–139
29. Carroli G, Belizan J (2000) Episiotomy for vaginal birth. Cochrane Database Syst Rev (1):CD000081
30. Christianson LM, Bovbjerg VE, McDavitt EC, Hullfish KL (2003) Risk factors for perineal injury during delivery. Am J Obstet Gynecol 189(1):255–260
31. Dudding TC, Vaizey CJ, Kamm MA (2008) Obstetric anal sphincter injury: incidence, risk factors, and management. Ann Surg 247(2):224–237
32. Fritel X, Schaal J, Fauconnier A, Bertrand V, Levet C, Pigne A (2008) Pelvic floor disorders four years after first delivery: a comparative study of restrictive versus systematic episiotomy. BJOG 115:247–252
33. Gee AS, Jones RS, Durdey P (2000) On line quantitative analysis of surface electromyography of the pelvic floor in patients with faecal incontinence. Br J Surg 87(6):814–818
34. Gregory WT, Lou JS, Simmons K, Clark AL (2008) Quantitative anal sphincter electromyography in primiparous women with anal incontinence. Am J Obstet Gynecol 198(5):550.e1–550.e6

35. Guise JM, Morris C, Osterwell P, Li H, Rosenberg D, Greenlick M (2007) Incidence of fecal incontinence after childbirth. Obstet Gynecol 109:281–288
36. McKinnie V, Swift SE, Wang W, Woodman P, O'Boyle A, Kahn M, Valley M, Bland D, Schaffer J (2005) The effect of pregnancy and mode of delivery on the prevalence of urinary and fecal incontinence. Am J Obstet Gynecol 193:512–517
37. Murphy D, Macleod M, Bahl R, Goyder K, Howarth L, Strachan B (2008) A randomized controlled trial of routine versus restrictive use of episiotomy at operative vaginal delivery: a multicenter Pilot study. BJOG 115(13):1695–1702; discussion 1702–3 (2008)
38. Nelson RL (2004) Epidemiology of faecal incontinence. Gastroenterology 126:3–7
39. Fitzgerald MP, Weber AM, Howden N, Cundiff GW, Brown MB (2007) Risk factors for anal sphincter tear during vaginal delivery. Obstet Gynecol 109(1):29–34
40. Handa VL, Blomquist JL, McDermott KC, Friedman S, Muñoz A (2012) Pelvic floor disorders after vaginal birth: effect of episiotomy, perineal laceration, and operative birth. Obstet Gynecol 119(2 Pt 1):233–239
41. Kudish B, Blackwell S, Mcneeley SG, Bujold E, Kruger M, Hendrix SL, Sokol R (2006) Operative vaginal delivery and midline episiotomy: a bad combination for the perineum. Am J Obstet Gynecol 195:749–754
42. Lewicky-Gaupp C, Hamilton Q, Ashton-Miller J, Huebner M, DeLancey JQ, Fenner DE (2009) Anal sphincter structure and function relationships in aging and fecal incontinence. Am J Obstet Gynecol 200(5):559
43. Oberwalder M, Dinnewitzer A, Baig MK, Thaler K, Cotman K, Nogueras JJ, Weiss EG, Efron J, Vernava AM, Wexner SD (2004) The association between late-onset fecal incontinence and obstetric anal sphincter defects. Arch Surg 139(4):429–432
44. Macmillan AK, Merrie AE, Marshall RJ, Parry BR (2004) The prevalence of fecal incontinence in community-dwelling adults: a systematic review of the literature. Dis Colon Rectum 47:1341–1349
45. Mellgren A, Jensen LL, Zetterstrom JP et al (1999) Long-term cost of fecal incontinence secondary to obstetric injuries. Dis Colon Rectum 42:857–867
46. Hartmann K, Meera Viswanathan M, Palmieri R, Gartlehner G, Thorp J, Lohr K (2005) Outcomes of routine episiotomy a systematic review. JAMA 293(17):2141–2148
47. Eason E, Labrecque M, Marcoux S, Mondor M (2002) Anal incontinence after childbirth. CMAJ 166(3):326–330
48. van Brummen HJ, Bruinse HW, van de Pol G, Heintz AP, van der Vaart CH (2006) Defecatory symptoms during and after the first pregnancy: prevalences and associated factors. Int Urogynecol J Pelvic Floor Dysfunct 17(3):224–230, Epub 2005 Aug 3
49. Tetzschner T, Sørensen M, Lose G, Christiansen J (1996) Anal and urinary incontinence in women with obstetric anal sphincter rupture. Br J Obstet Gynaecol 103(10):1034–1040
50. Kamm MA (2003) Faecal incontinence. BMJ 327:1299–1300
51. Deutekom M, Terra MP, Dobben AC, Dijkgraaf MG, Felt-Bersma RJ, Stoker J, Bossuyt PM (2005) Selecting an outcome measure for evaluating treatment in fecal incontinence. Dis Colon Rectum 48(12):2294–2301
52. Sung VW, Rogers ML, Myers DL, Akbari HM, Clark MA (2007) National trends and costs of surgical treatment for female fecal incontinence. Am J Obstet Gynecol 197(6):652.e1–652.e5
53. Amorim M, Franca-Neto A, Leal N, Melo F, Maia S, Alve J (2014) Is it possible to never perform episiotomy during vaginal delivery ? Obstet Gynecol 123(Suppl 1):38S. doi:10.1097/01.AOG.0000447311 4.51968.54
54. Bharucha AE, Zinsmeister AR, Locke GR, Seide BM, McKeon K, Schleck CD, Melton LJ (2005) Prevalence and burden of fecal incontinence: a population-based study in women. Gastroenterology 129:42–49
55. Weber AM (2004) The perspective of a gynecologist on treatment-related research for fecal incontinence in women. Gastroenterology 126:S169–S171
56. Pirro N, Sastre B, Sielezneff IJ (2007) What are the risk factors of anal incontinence after vaginal delivery? J Chir (Paris) 144(3):197–202, Review. French

57. South MM, Stinnet SS, Sanders DB, Weidner AC (2009) Levator ani denervation and reinnervation six months after childbirth. Am J Obstet Gynecol 200(5):519.e1–519.e7
58. Woolley RJ (1995) Benefits and risks of episiotomy: a review of the English-language literature since 1980. Part I and Part II. Obstet Gynecol Surv 50:806–835
59. Wunderlich M, Swash M (1993) The overlapping innervation of the two sides of the external anal sphincter by the pudendal nerves. J Neurol Sci 59:97–109

8 Sexual Function After Delivery

Stefano Salvatore, Anna Redaelli, Ilaria Baini,
and Massimo Candiani

Few studies have been carried out on post-partum sexual function; in fact, little is known concerning postnatal sexual dysfunctions related to childbirth in various ways and/or obstetric risk factors. Sexual dysfunction is a multifaceted disorder that occurs frequently and concerns various aspects of sexuality:

- Sexual desire disorders that are often related to the hypo efficiency of the pelvic floor, which occurs post-partum
- Sexual arousal disorders due to the vaginal dryness and poor lubrication typical of breastfeeding women
- Orgasmic disorders related to hypotonia due to childbirth which causes pain and inability to reach orgasm
- Superficial dyspareunia (pain during penetration)

In general, the prevalence of post-partum sexual dysfunction ranges between 22 and 50 %. In a study carried out by Odar et al., at a 6-month post-partum follow-up, 22.2 % reported having sexual problems due to vaginal pain (18.8 % due to lacerations) or blood loss (15.6 %) [1]. According to Barrett et al., only 15 % of women suffering from post-partum sexual dysfunctions report the problem to their doctor [2].

Pelvic floor traumas are often related to sexual dysfunction and are associated with the following risk factors: advanced maternal age, low BMI with operative delivery, prolonged second stage of labour, foetal head circumference and episiotomy.

S. Salvatore (✉) • A. Redaelli • I. Baini • M. Candiani
Department of Obstetrics & Gynecology, San Raffaele University, Milan, Italy

D. Riva, G. Minini (eds.), *Childbirth-Related Pelvic Floor Dysfunction: Risk Factors, Prevention, Evaluation, and Treatment*,
DOI 10.1007/978-3-319-18197-4_8

8.1 Time Required for Resuming Sexual Intercourse

The time required for resuming sexual intercourse after childbirth varies from woman to woman and is influenced by many factors. Signorello et al. studied the time required for resuming sexual intercourse following childbirth for a cohort of 626 women who had vaginal delivery with or without episiotomy and vaginal tears. After 6 months all women included in the study had resumed having sexual intercourse regardless of the level of laceration. Women with lower grades of laceration (grades I and II) had resumed having sexual intercourse on average 7.1 weeks post-partum while women with higher grades of lacerations (grades III and IV) had resumed sexual intercourse on average 9.3 months post-partum. Moreover patients aged ≥35 years of age resumed having sexual intercourse on average 2.5 weeks later than women aged <25 years of age. Black women resumed having sexual intercourse on average 1.2 weeks earlier than white women. Breastfeeding women resumed having sexual intercourse 0.8 weeks earlier than non-breastfeeding women [3].

In the study by Brubaker et al., the percentage of women who began having sexual intercourse at 6 months post-partum was approximately 90 %. The resumption of sexual intercourse was slightly longer for women with 3rd and 4th degree perineal tears and women who underwent caesarean sections than women with vaginal delivery [4].

8.2 Dyspareunia

Dyspareunia post-partum is a fairly common problem. In a study carried out by Odal et al. approximately 62 % of women who resumed having sexual intercourse 6 month after childbirth reported pain [1].

The study by Basksu et al. shows that women who undergo a paramedian episiotomy have an increase in the level of pain at 6 months post-partum compared to women who have elective caesarean sections [5]. The same result is reported by Safarinejad et al. [6].

This finding is in agreement with the study by Klein et al. which showed that the first-time mothers who had elective caesarean sections had better-toned pelvic floors than women who had a delivery. This leads many women to prefer giving birth by caesarean section than vaginal delivery. Besides the pain, it appears to have a predominant effect on the total FSFI score [7] as well as on sexual satisfaction.

Among women who had a delivery, the women with 3rd and 4th grade vaginal tears reported feeling more pain than the patients with intact perineum which decreased at 3 and 6 months post-partum in both cases [3]. Moreover, women who underwent episiotomy reported feeling more pain at their first sexual intercourse after childbirth than women who with a spontaneous perineal lacerations.

According to Brubaker et al., it is estimated that 20 % of women report feeling pain during sexual intercourse at 3 months post-partum and one fifth of them feel pain after 6 months [4].

8.3 Sexual Desire

It is well known that sexual desire is still reduced 1 year after giving birth and that sexual intercourse is less frequent [2, 8], yet it is difficult to determine if this is due to psychological or physical issues.

There are also organic causes which may cause low sexual desire: low levels of oestrogen which reduce vaginal lubrication and lead to less congestion of blood vessels, high prolactin levels especially when breastfeeding which leads to mood changes and lastly a drop in androgen which is ultimately responsible for loss of sexual desire.

Waterstone et al. states that the type of delivery or episiotomy are not the only factors responsible for loss of desire and that other issues may come into play: lack of interest in one's partner, fear of getting pregnant again and fear of feeling genital discomfort [9].

Safarinejad argues that women who undergo operative deliveries, emergency caesarean sections or episiotomies are more prone to sexual desire disorders compared to patients who have eutocic deliveries without episiotomy or elective caesarean sections [6].

8.4 Sexual Arousal, Orgasm, Lubrification and Sexual Satisfaction

Sexual arousal, orgasm and lubrication undergo some changes after delivery. The reason for these changes is difficult to define. They could be both psychological and physical. Safarinejad et al. reported that both women who deliver vaginally and by caesarean section referred a decline in sexual arousal, more important in women after operative delivery. Lubrication disorders are associated with hypoestrogenic state typical of breastfeeding that brings to vaginal dryness [6]. Sexual satisfaction is reduced in post-partum women and it does not depend on the mode of delivery; it improves with time [6].

8.5 Partner Sexual Satisfaction

Sexual dysfunctions do not involve only women; they also affected women's partners. Safarinejad et al. reported male partners' sexual dysfunctions related to the mode of delivery of their women. Partners of women who underwent instrumental delivery suffered of erectile dysfunction more frequently than partners of women who deliver vaginally or by caesarean section. Orgasm, sexual arousal and sexual satisfaction were not affected by women's mode of delivery. Partners of women who underwent an elective caesarean section were more satisfied after 3 months post-partum [6]. According to Gungor et al., vaginal penetration perception was changed in the post-partum period both in women than in men [10].

8.6 Psychological Argument

Psychology plays an important role in the development of sexual dysfunction. Sexuality is an important issue of couple life. Culture, emotion and religion affect couple's post-partum life. The birth of a baby could disrupt a couple's balance, and it depends on the cultural environment. The birth of a baby brings some changes on the physical aspects, in particular on genitalia. Women who underwent episiotomy refer pain and consequently fear of resumption of sexual intercourse.

Many post-partum women suffer of some sexual dysfunction, such as loss of sexual desire, dyspareunia, loss of lubrication, pain at orgasm, vaginal bleeding and vaginal aching. From pregnancy to delivery, a woman's body undergoes some changes that can bring psychological consequences. After delivery, women suffer physical and emotional dysfunctions that can worsen over time. Sexual dysfunction could bring to women and women's partners unhappiness. In the post-partum, women could feel guilty of being a bad but healthy and happy mother and partner because of tiredness, anxiety, depression and poor quality of life.

Financial and relational problems are associated with a high incidence of psychological symptoms; this emphasizes the importance of a social environment and a good couple life of post-partum women.

References

1. Odar E, Wandabwa J, Kiondo P (2003) Sexual practices of women within six months of childbirth in Mulago Hospital. Uganda. Afr Health Sci 3(3):117–123
2. Barret G, Pendry E, Peacock J, Victor C, Thaker R, Manyonda I (2000) Women's sexual health after childbirth. Br J Obstet Gynecol 107:186–195
3. Signorello LB, Harlow BL, Chekos AK, Repke JT (2001) Postpartum sexual functioning and its relationship to perineal trauma: a retrospective cohort study of primiparous women. Am J Obstet Gynecol 184:881–890
4. Brubaker L, Handa VL, Bradly CS, Connoly AM, Moalli P, Brown MB et al (2008) Sexual function 6 months after first delivery. Obstet Gynecol 111(5):1040–1044
5. Baksu B, Davas I, Agar E, Akyol A, Varolan A (2007) The effect of mode of delivery on postpartum sexual functioning in primiparous women. Int Urogynecol J Pelvic Flood Dysfunct 18(4):401–406
6. Safarinejad MR, Kolahi AA, Hosseini L (2009) The effect of mode of delivery on the quality of life, sexual function, and sexual satisfaction in primiparous women and their housband. J Sex Med 6(6):1645–1667
7. Klein M, Gauthier R, Jorgensen S, Robbins J, Kaczorowski J, Franco ED et al (1994) Relationship of episioromy to perineal trauma and morbidity, sexual function, and pelvic floor relaxation. Am J Obstet Gynecol 171:591–598
8. Morof D, Barret G, Peacock J, Victor C, Mandyonda I (2003) Postnatal depression and sexual health after childbirth. Obstet Gynecol 102:1318–1325
9. Waterstone M, Wolfe C, Hooper R, Bewley S (2003) Postnatal morbidity after childbirth and severe obstetric morbidity. Br J Obstet Gynecol 110:128–133
10. Gungor S, Baser I, Ceyhan T, Karasahin E, Kilic S (2008) Does mode of delivery affect sexual functioning of the man partner? J Sex Med 5(1):155–163

The Controversial Role of Episiotomy 9

Diego Riva

9.1 Introduction

Episiotomy is the term used for identifying the surgical cutting, made usually with scissors, of vaginal and perineal tissues, beginning at the level of the posterior fourchette or few millimetres lateral to it, during the second stage of labour, in order to enlarge the vulvar introitus: this manoeuvre can avoid an excessive trauma to that area and accelerate the delivery in case of fetal distress. Anatomical structures that can be involved are vaginal wall, bulbo-cavernous, superficial and deep transverse perineal muscles. Lesions of external and internal anal sphincters or of pubo-rectalis muscle can occur if deeper structures are interested during episiotomy itself or as a consequence of unexpected lacerations. It was performed for the first time in 1742 by C. Ould to prevent a serious perineal damage, but the term was introduced only by C Braun in 1857. Its use in Northern American literature was described in 1852 by Tagliaferro as a part of the obstetric assistance in pre-eclamptic women. Beginning from the 20s of the last century, episiotomy gained popularity as a method to reduce fetal trauma in complicated deliveries in primiparae, and in the following years it was used even to prevent severe maternal sequelae as deep vaginal tears or anal disruptions.

Since the 1980s, it became widely adopted by midwives both in the USA and in Europe, and it was considered as a part of the routine birth assistance, even if a clear demonstration of its efficacy to reduce *perineal damage* was not reached. Beginning from the 90s, a great variety of randomized study was conducted to investigate the protective or the negative role of episiotomy as regards a series of consequences of *vaginal birth*, that is perineal pain, dyspareunia, impaired innervations of muscular tissues, urinary and anal incontinence. More recently, many studies focused on the

D. Riva
Department of Obstetric and Gynecologic, Clinica S. Pio X, Milan, Italy
e-mail: diriva@tiscali.it

D. Riva, G. Minini (eds.), *Childbirth-Related Pelvic Floor Dysfunction: Risk Factors, Prevention, Evaluation, and Treatment*,
DOI 10.1007/978-3-319-18197-4_9

pros and cons of a restrictive use of episiotomy or a particular type of episiotomy, in relationship to the long-term sequelae of perineal trauma: among them anal sphincter injuries (OASIS) represent undoubtedly a major concern after vaginal birth as they are the commonest cause of faecal incontinence.

From a general point of view, the following risk factors for 3rd or 4th degree tears were reported by P. Aukee et al. [1]: primiparity (OR: 5.42), vacuum extraction (OR 2.98), parietal presentation (OR 5.64) and neonatal weight >4,000 g (OR 3.01). As regards episiotomy, they suggested that it had a protective role against perineal tears.

In this chapter, we will debate some related questions. Which is the best policy: a restrictive or a routine use of episiotomy? In which cases episiotomy may have a protective or a negative action? How episiotomy must be performed to be really protective? Is there any difference between primiparae and multiparae or during operative vaginal birth? Which is the role of caesarean section as regards pelvic floor integrity?

9.2 Routine or Restrictive Use of Episiotomy

Nowadays, OMS recommends that episiotomy should be performed not routinely, but only when necessary; following these suggestions it ought to be used in no more than 5–10 % of deliveries [2]. Despite that, it represents all over the world the most widely performed operation during delivery, always without obtaining an informed consent, and in Europe the average rate is reported to be about 30 %, reaching the rate of 80 % in many obstetrical departments. There is a great variability of rates in different European countries, ranging from 9.7 % in Sweden, 22 % in Finland, 13–25 % in Great Britain, to 30–49 % in France, 58 % in Italy and finally 87.3 % in Spain. In Central and South America, its rates are shown to be about 95 %.

Therefore, the pros and cons of a *restrictive use of episiotomy* are still now very often debated by most researchers. The supporters of routine episiotomy claim that it prevents from uncontrolled tears and deep lacerations of pelvic musculature, but their arguments are far from being fully clarified: first of all the consequences of 1st and 2nd spontaneous lacerations are practically absent [3] and the most feared deep lacerations that are followed by long-term dysfunctions as urinary and/or anal incontinence are not always avoided by episiotomy.

Other studies examined the risk of *4th degree tears* (4° DT) in different institutes, where routine or selective mediolateral episiotomies (MLE) were performed: the rate of tears were globally equal (1.6 %), being comprised between 0 and 6.6 % in both groups, the rates of MLE being on the contrary comprised between 51 and 100 % [4–9] (Table 9.1).

In 2011, Raisanen et al. [10] examined the consequences of different delivery policies in Finland on the risks of anal sphincter ruptures: they concluded that episiotomy was a weak protective factor (OR 0.82) only in primiparous patients but not in multiparous ones (OR 2.86) and that therefore a high rate of episiotomy had probably to be preferred in primiparae. They also observed that episiotomy in multiparous women was performed frequently only if a risk factor for OASIS was present.

Table 9.1 Risk of 4th degree tears (4° DT)

Ref n°	Pts n°	Selective MLE (4°DT%)	Routine MLE (4°DT%)	OR
5	181	0	5.6	0.12
6	2,606	1.2	1.5	0.78
7	698	6.6	6.6	1
8	881	0.45	0	7.32
9	1,000	0.8	0.2	3.36
Total	5,366	1.6	1.6	0.91

Table 9.2 The impact of episiotomy on urinary incontinence after 3 months or 3 years with routine episiotomy (RE) or selective episiotomy (SE)

	3 months RE	SE	3 years RE	SE
UI	4 %	6 %	8 %	9 %
UI	18 %	17 %	Not rep	Not rep

As regards urinary incontinence after 3 months and 3 years after delivery, two studies [7–9] did not find any difference between a selective or a routine use of mediolateral episiotomy (Table 9.2).

Even the overview published by Myers-Helfgott et al. [11] underlines the same concept.

Therefore, as for this topic, in conclusion we agree with the affirmation that there is little evidence to support routine episiotomy in modern obstetric practice.

9.3 How Episiotomy Must Be Performed

A main question regards how episiotomy is performed, because it has a fundamental influence on anatomical structures that can be involved not only directly during the episiotomy itself, but also as regards the possibility of vaginal tears in other areas: this fact can occur if vaginal introitus is not enlarged enough by episiotomy to allow the passage of the fetus without creating other lesions, or if the incision is involuntarily widened creating a damage in the deeper structures. We must remember that the three variations of episiotomy are medial, a midline incision from the fourchette toward the anal canal, mediolateral, that begins at the midline and is directed laterally reaching an angle between 40° and 60° to the left or to the right of the anal canal, and lateral in which the incision begins laterally from the midline at 4–5 or 7–8 o'clock.

Following the classification and *standardization of episiotomies* published by Kalis et al. in 2012 [12], they can therefore be distinguished by type, origin of the initial incision and direction of the cut. Therefore, in every patient, the point of origin in relationship with the posterior fourchette, the angle from the midline, the length of the cut and the distance from the anal canal ought to be calculated (Fig. 9.1).

In the vast majority of obstetrical wards, only the midline and the mediolateral incisions are used.

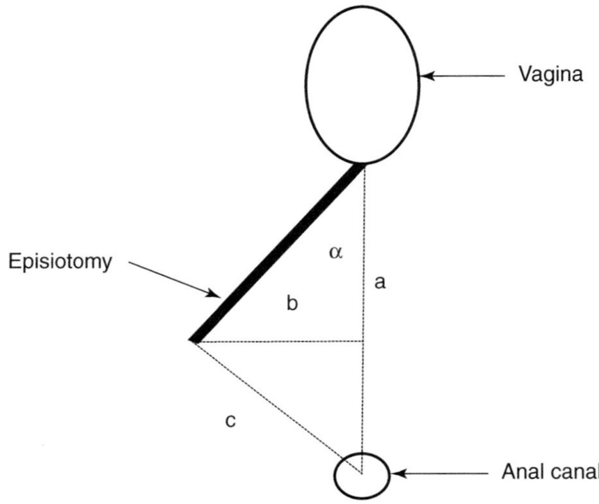

Fig. 9.1 Graphic representation of episiotomy. Capture. (*a*) Midline between vagina and anal canal. (*b*) Distance between the end of MLE and a. (*c*) Distance between the end of MLE and anus. (α) Angle of MLE

The right way in which it must be performed (midline versus mediolateral) is a key point and is widely debated: for example, Coat et al. [13] reported that midline episiotomy was followed by anal laceration in 11.6 % of women, while only 2 % experienced such complication after mediolateral episiotomy. Other authors reported that the OR for complete lacerations after midline episiotomy ranged between 1.08 and 22 in spontaneous vaginal deliveries [14–16]. Studies evaluating the episiotomy technique showed that the angle is significantly associated with OASIS: Injuries occurred more frequently when the angle is inferior to 40° [17, 18].

In a very sophisticated study, Stedenfeldt et al. [19] in 2012 examined two groups of women who had had episiotomy or not as regarded the occurrence of OASIS: they showed that the risk of sphincter laceration decreased by 70 % by each 5.5 mm. increase in episiotomy depth, and by 56 % for every 4.5 mm increase in the distance from the midline.

Despite that, midline episiotomy is still widely performed because it appears more physiologic; it is considered easier to heal and is reported to cause less perineal pain or long-term dyspareunia. In our opinion, midline episiotomy should be almost abandoned, as it may be very dangerous: it has to be performed only by well-trained midwives, in non-operative deliveries and with fetuses with normal weight.

We must underline that the timing of episiotomy is also very important, as it must be done before the occurrence of any nervous stretching or anal sphincter disruption.

9.4 Episiotomy in Operative Delivery

A different question regards *operative vaginal deliveries*, in which episiotomy could be more effective in avoiding OASIS.

Even for this point, opinions are often different. In 2008, Murphy et al. [20] reported about the effects of routine versus restricted use of episiotomy in operative vaginal delivery, in a randomized trial, but their results, regarding 317 operative vaginal deliveries, were inconclusive: they did not find any evidence that routine episiotomy was better than a restrictive one in preventing 3rd or 4th degree tears; anal sphincter tears were 8.1 % with routine episiotomy in comparison with 10.9 % with restrictive use: No statistical difference was reached, but this result was probably negative because their samples were too small.

On the other hand, a larger retrospective study published by deLeeuw et al. [21] in 2008 showed that episiotomy appeared highly protective against anal sphincter tears both in forceps and in vacuum births: they demonstrated that the risk of anal incontinence after a complete perineal tear was lower if the patient had a mediolateral episiotomy (12 % vs. 46 %): this fact could be related also to the protective effect against neurological lesions.

The same opinion was expressed by de Vogel et al. [22]: in a very large study, they found that when MLE was performed, the risk of developing OASIS after operative vaginal delivery was decreased by sixfold (3.3 % vs. 15.6 %).

These dramatic differences may be related to different clinical behaviours in the timing of episiotomy or to its technique or indeed to the classification of anal tears. The comparison among the three studies underlines that the argument is not well clarified and that many confounding elements may contribute to different results, but the vast majority of authors agree that a MLE must be performed in operative vaginal deliveries. As a matter of fact, in order to prevent anal sphincter tears, a strict cooperation between the doctor and the midwife is required during operative delivery to ensure the best perineal support and the right timing of episiotomy.

9.5 Pelvic Floor Damage and the Opportunity for Caesarean Section

It is well known that vaginal birth represents the major cause of *anal incontinence* (AI): even if lacerations of anal sphincter are uncommon, they represent a major complication of delivery with high percentages of subsequent faecal incontinence and/or defecatory problems: as a matter of fact, the incidence of AI following 3rd or 4th degree tears is reported as ranging from 7 to 56 %. We have already underlined that undoubtedly median episiotomy is to be considered at higher risk of anal sphincter tear, as reported even in recent studies [19]. The damage of anal sphincter can be due both to a direct lesion, eventually not completely sutured after delivery, and/or to denervation, following stretching or laceration of pudendal nerve terminations. Beginning from the studies of Snooks et al. in the 80s [23], denervation of the pelvic floor after vaginal delivery was fully demonstrated in about 80 % of women.

Stretching to pudendal nerve can lead to cumulative damages to pelvic floor, so that muscular denervation, atrophy, fibrosis and finally impaired function and defective organ support usually follow. As a matter of fact, up to 25 % of primiparous women experience small degrees of AI post-partum and one third show some aspects of anal sphincter injury. In most women, faecal incontinence resolves spontaneously, but at the age of 65 it affects about 13 per 1,000 women.

The study performed by Casey et al. [24] involving 10,643 primiparous women showed that episiotomy represented an odd factor for post-partum anal incontinence (OR 1.7) and for any type of urinary incontinence (both urge and stress types).

Other authors reported that after instrumental vaginal delivery the risk of anal incontinence is increased with an OR of 1.94–7.2; the risk of urinary incontinence appears to be increased with an OR of 1.81, while the frequency of urgency is increased of 4.2 times [21, 22].

A very intriguing question regards the widened request for *elective caesarean section* that is often based on this fact.

One hundred and four caesarean sections performed for emergency, 80 elective ones and 100 vaginal births with no perineal laceration were compared by Mira Lai et al. [25]: they found that the risk of anal incontinence was similar among the three groups.

A comparison between nulliparous women and patients submitted to CS showed that the rates of anal gas incontinence, faecal incontinence, stress urinary incontinence and overactive bladder (OAB) were respectively: 5 and 9 % (gas incontinence), 2 and 4 % (faecal incontinence), 11 and 18 % (SUI) and 4 and 6 % (OAB), showing that CS does not have a complete protective action against pelvic floor deterioration during pregnancy [26]. Examining *pelvic floor strength* after childbirth, T. Sigurdardottir, K. Bo et al. [27] found a significant reduction in PFM strength ($p<0.0001$) and endurance ($p<0.0001$) in all participants to their study after the first childbirth. The reduction in strength was 20.1 hPa (CI:16.2; 24.1), 31.4 hPa (CI: 7.4; 55.2) 5.2 hPa (CI: −6.6; 17.0) in the normal vaginal, instrumental vaginal and acute caesarean groups, respectively. The difference was significant between normal vaginal and acute caesarean birth ($p=0.028$) and between instrumental vaginal and acute caesarean birth ($p=0.003$). They concluded that PFM strength is significantly reduced after vaginal delivery, both normal and instrumental, 6–12 weeks postpartum, and that acute caesarean section resulted in significantly less muscle strength reduction.

The effect of pregnancy and mode of delivery on *pelvic floor muscle function* (PFMF) was prospectively evaluated also by K. Elenskaia et al. [28] by means of a subjective method (Oxford scale) and an objective analysis (perineometry). An assessment of PFMF was performed at 20 and 36 weeks of gestation and at 14 weeks and 12 months after delivery. The resting pressure (RP) and the maximum squeeze pressure (MSP) were recorded. Results showed that between the 403 women (182 nulliparous and 221 multiparous) recruited, 294 (73 %) delivered vaginally and 92 (23 %) by caesarean section: RP and MSP improved significantly ($p<0.01$) during pregnancy. After childbirth, a significant decrease in PFMF was demonstrated that recovered completely by 1 year in the majority of women. They concluded that a physiological increment in PFMF during pregnancy appears to be common and that the pelvic floor weakens temporarily after childbirth but contractility appears to recover by 1 year, irrespective of the mode of delivery.

In a recently published study, Cescon, Riva et al. [29] reported the results of an EMG analysis of external anal sphincter fibres and motor units before and after vaginal birth: They demonstrated that, in comparison with CS and deliveries

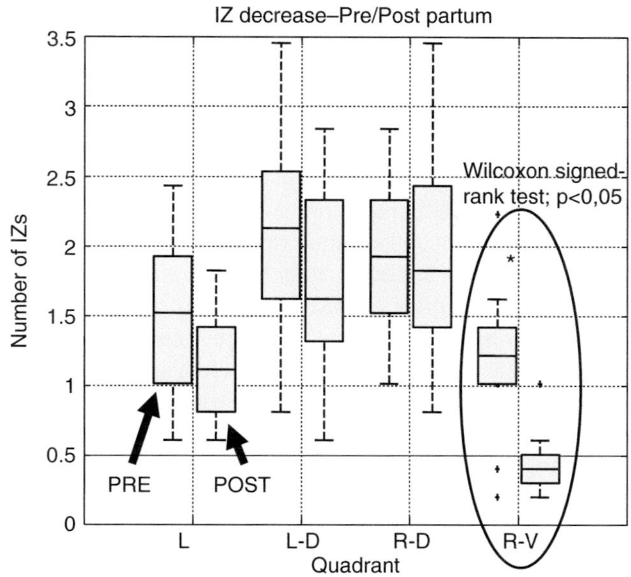

Fig. 9.2 Innervation zone analysis after MLE in the 4 quadrants

performed without an episiotomy, MLE is significantly followed by external *anal sphincter denervation* due to a reduction of innervations zones (IZ) in the side (Right Ventral Quadrant) where it has been performed (Fig. 9.2).

Dupuis et al. [4] demonstrated that after a CS the risk of developing urinary incontinence was reduced (OR = 0.62; 95 % IC: 0.41–0.93), while there was no benefit regarding anal incontinence both for gas (OR = 1.10; 95 % IC [0.79–1.54]) and for stool (OR = 0.54; 95 % IC [0.18–1.62]). This study may suffer from the bias due to the fact that it was based on an "intention to treat" analysis, so that only 57 % of women in the group of vaginal delivery underwent really to a vaginal birth. Beginning from 1993, Sultan et al. [30] as part of a study on delivery-related anal sphincter damage found that 10 % of 127 women who delivered vaginally had anal incontinence (including incontinence of flatus) or urgency 6–8 weeks later. This sample, however, was small and may not have been representative since it included only those women who agreed to have a complete anal and perineal assessment. They also showed that if CS was performed during labour, latency times of pudendal nerves were higher 6 weeks after the first delivery in comparison to elective CS and that there was a 35 % of echographic defect in anal sphincter. In a more recent study [31], they found that echographic defect ranged between 9 and 53 % and anal incontinence between 0 and 17 %: It meant that about 50 % of women with echographic defect were asymptomatic.

In the same way, Mac Arthur et al. [32] showed that among 113 women submitted to emergency CS, 6 suffered from anal or urge faecal incontinence, confirming that at the time of CS neurological lesions were already present. In their study, 36 women (4 %) developed new faecal incontinence after the index birth, 22 of whom had unresolved symptoms. Twenty-seven had symptoms several times a week, yet only five consulted a doctor. Among vaginal deliveries, forceps and vacuum extraction were the only independent risk factors: 12 (33 %) of those with new incontinence had an instrumental delivery compared with 114 (14 %) of the 847 women who had never had faecal incontinence. Six of those with incontinence had an emergency caesarean section but none became incontinent after elective sections.

They concluded that faecal incontinence as an immediate consequence of childbirth is more common than previously realized, and that medical attention is rarely sought. Forceps and vacuum extraction deliveries represent risk factors, with no protection demonstrated by emergency caesarean sections. Identification and treatment represent a great priority.

Apart from the risks related to surgery and post-operative complications, we can conclude that CS is not always protective against pelvic floor damage and that its risks must be balanced against fetal well-being and the risk of maternal perineal lesions.

Taking finally into account other considerations, we can remember that different perineal techniques and interventions are suggested to prevent perineal trauma. These interventions include perineal massage, warm compresses and perineal management techniques.

Some authors reported about the protective action of *perineal massage* during pregnancy in primiparas, just similarly to perineal support and close observation during delivery (Pirhonen et al. [33] – Samuelsson et al. [34]). On the other hand, other authors do not completely agree with these affirmations (E. Eason et al. [35]) An interesting question regards the methods of delivery in women who had experienced a third-degree tear during their first delivery: following the study of Fynes et al. [36], episiotomy seems to increase the risk of a further tear.

Cassado et al. [37] investigated with 4D ultrasound if episiotomy could be protective against *levator ani avulsion* but their results were not statistically significant, probably because their sample of 194 patients was too small.

As regards dyspareunia, it was reported by 24 % of women after delivery [38], but the role of episiotomy is controversial on this matter.

The last topic is related to a woman who has sustained a sphincter injury during her first delivery. Subsequent deliveries by CS are commonly suggested, while a late recourse to CS during an advanced labour is not considered protective against perineal nervous trauma. In this matter, the role of episiotomy is therefore not relevant.

Conclusions

The aim to avoid long-lasting damages of pelvic floor structures after vaginal delivery, affecting severely quality of life, must be our goal. The analysis of literature indicates that episiotomy is not to be suggested in a routine fashion. If demonstrated risk factors are present (e.g. an operative vaginal delivery or a high weight baby), mediolateral episiotomy represents undoubtedly the best choice. Elective caesarean section is not protective against pelvic floor dysfunction, because pregnancy itself can affect muscular, nervous and connective structures before delivery; the role of denervation and subsequent re-innervation are very intriguing topics in this field.

References

1. Aukee P, Sundstrom H, Kairaluoma MV (2006) The role of mediolateral episiotomy during labour: analysis of risk factors for obstetric anal sphincter rears. Acta Obstet Gynecol Scand 85(7):856–860
2. Carroli G, Mignini L (2012) Episiotomy for vaginal birth. Cochrane Database Syst Rev 2:CD000081
3. Fitzpatrick M, O'Herlihy C (2001) The effect of labour and delivery on the pelvic floor. Best Pract Res Obstet Gynecol 15(1):63–79
4. Dupuis O, Madelenat P, Rudigoz RC et al (2004) Fecal and urinary incontinence after delivery: risk factors and prevention. Gynecol Obstet Fertil 32:540–548
5. Harrison RF, Brennan M, North PM et al (1984) Is routine episiotomy necessary? Br Med J 30:1971–1975
6. Group AETC Routine vs. selective episiotomy: a randomized controlled trial (1993) Lancet 342:1517–1518
7. Klein MC, Gauthier RJ, Jorgensen SH et al (1992) Does episiotomy prevent perineal trauma and pelvic floor relaxation? Online J Curr Clin Trials
8. Flint C, Poulengeris P (1987) In: Heinemann W (ed) The "Know your midwife" report. London
9. Sleep J, Grant A (1987) West Berkshire perineal management trial: three year follow up. Br Med J 26:749–751
10. Raisanen S, Vehvilainen-Julkunen K, Gissler M et al (2011) High episiotomy rates protect from obstetric and sphincter ruptures: a birth register-study on delivery intervention policies in Finland. Scan J Pub Health 39(5):457–463
11. Myers-Helfgott M, Helfgott A (1999) Routine use of episiotomy in modern obstetrics- should it be performed? Obstet Gynecol Clin North Am 26:305–325
12. Kalis V, Landsmanova J, Bednarova B et al (2001) Evaluation of the incision angle of mediolateral episiotomy at 60 degrees. Int J Gynaecol Obstet 112(3):220–224
13. Coats PM, Chan KK, Wilkins M, Beard RJ (1980) A comparison between midline and mediolateral episiotomies. Br J Obstet Gynecol 87:408–413
14. Anthony S, Buitendijk SE, Zondervan KT et al (1994) Episiotomies and the occurrence of severe perineal lacerations. Br J Obstet Gynaecol 101:1064–1067
15. Klein MC, Gauthier RJ, Robbins JM (1994) Relationship of episiotomy to perineal trauma and morbidity, sexual dysfunction, and pelvic floor relaxation. Am J Obstet Gynecol 171:591–598
16. Borgatta L, Piening SL, Cohen WR (1989) Association of episiotomy and delivery position with deep perineal laceration during spontaneous delivery in nulliparous women. Am J Obstet Gynecol 160:294–297
17. Andrews V, Thakar R, Sultan AH, Jones P (2005) Are mediolateral episiotomies actually mediolateral? BJOG 112:1156–1158
18. Bodner-Adler B, Bodner K, Kaider A et al (2001) Risk factors for third degree perineal tears in vaginal delivery, with an analysis of episiotomy types. J Reprod Med 46:752–756
19. Stedenfeld M, Pirhonen J, Blix E et al (2012) Episiotomy characteristics and risks for obstetric anal sphincter injuries: a case controlled study. BJOG 119:724–730
20. Murphy DJ, Macleod M, Bahl R et al (2008) A randomized controlled trial of routine versus restrictive use of episiotomy at operative vaginal delivery: a multicenter pilot study. BJOG 115:1695–1703
21. deLeeuw JW, de Wit C, Kuijken JP et al (2008) Mediolateral episiotomy reduces the risk for anal sphincter injury during operative vaginal delivery. BJOG 115:104–108
22. deVogel J, van der Leeuw-van Beek A, Dirk Gietelink D et al (2012) The effect of a mediolateral episiotomy during operative vaginal delivery on the risk of developing obstetrical anal sphincter injuries. Am J Obstet Gynecol 2012;206:404.e1–404.e5
23. Snooks SJ, Setchell M et al (1984) Injury to innèrvations of pelvic floor sphincter musculature in childbirth. Lancet 2:546–550

24. Casey BM, Schaffer JI, Bloom SL et al (2005) Obstetric antecedents for postpartum pelvic floor dysfunction. Am J Obstet Gynecol 192:1655–1662
25. Lal M, Mann CH, Callender R et al (2003) Does cesarean delivery prevent anal incontinence? Obstet Gynecol 101:305–312
26. Peyrat L, Haillot O, Bruyere F et al (2002) Prevalence and risk factors of urinary incontinence in young and middle-aged women. BJU Int 89:61–66
27. Sigurdardottir T, Steingrimsdottir T et al (2011) Pelvic floor muscle function before and after first childbirth. Int Urogynecol J 192:1518–1519
28. Elenskaia K, Thakar R et al (2013) The effect of pregnancy and childbirth on pelvic muscle function. Int Urogynecol J 24(6):927–937
29. Cescon C, Riva D, Začesta V et al (2014) Effect of vaginal delivery on external anal sphincter muscle innervation pattern evaluated with multichannel surface EMG (Results of the multicenter study TASI-2). Int Urogynecol J. doi:10.1007/s00192-014-2375-0
30. Sultan AH, Kamm MA, Hudson CN et al (1993) Anal sphincter disruption during vaginal delivery. NEJM 329(26):1905–1911
31. Sultan AH, Monga AK (1997) Anal and urinary incontinence in women with obstetric anal sphincter rupture. BJOG 104(6):754–755
32. MacArthur C, Bick DE, Keighley MRB (1997) Fecal incontinence after childbirth. BJOG 104:46–50
33. Pirhonen JP, Grenman SE, Haadem K et al (1998) Frequency of anal sphincter rupture at delivery in Sweden and Finland – result of difference in manual help to the baby's head. Acta Obstet Gynecol Scand 77:974–977
34. Samuelsson E, Ladfors L, Wennerholm UB et al (2000) Anal sphincters tears: prospective study of obstetric risk factors. Br J Obstet Gynecol 107:926–931
35. Eason E, Labrecque M, Wells G, Feldman P (2000) Preventing perineal trauma during childbirth: a systematic review. Obstet Gynecol 95:464–471
36. Fynes M, Donnelly V, Behan M et al (1999) Effect on second vaginal delivery on anorectal physiology and faecal continence: a prospective study. Lancet 354:983–986
37. Cassado J, Pessarrodona A, Rodriguez-Carballeira M et al (2013) Does episiotomy protect against injury of the levator ani in normal vaginal delivery? Neurourol Urodyn 33(8):1212–6. doi:10.1002/nau.22488
38. Serati M, Salvatore S, Khullar V et al (2008) Prospective study to assess risk factors for pelvic floor dysfunction after delivery. Acta Obstet Gynecol Scand 87(3):313–318

Perineal Care During Pregnancy, Delivery, and Postpartum

10

Giuseppe Ettore, Gabriella Torrisi, and Sebastiana Ferraro

10.1 Introduction

Pregnancy and *vaginal childbirth* are often associated with neuromuscular and soft tissue injuries to the pelvic floor resulting in significant short-term and long-term morbidity [1–3]. Morbidity is more significant after third- and fourth-degree perineal tears and the rates of trauma are higher in nulliparous women [4].

Short-term morbidity includes pain and painful sex (dyspareunia) which impairs normal intercourse. Twenty percent of women who postpartum perineal trauma still have pain at 8 weeks [5], and 7–9 % report *pain* at 3 months [6]. Painful sex following vaginal delivery is reported by 30 % of women at 6 months [7]. Women who sustain severe perineal trauma reported more pain 7 weeks after delivery than those with minor trauma; however, this difference was no longer present by 3 months postpartum [8]. The long-term maternal morbidity results in female pelvic floor dysfunctions (PFD), including *urinary incontinence* (UI), *anal incontinence* (AI), and *pelvic organ prolapse* (POP).

After vaginal delivery around 15% of women develop stress urinary incontinence [9–11], 8 % experience incontinence of stool and 45 % suffer involuntary escape of flatus following anal sphincter damage even after injury recognition and repair [12, 13]. Six months postpartum stage 2 pelvic organ prolapse was noted in 18 % of primiparous women who delivered vaginally compared with 7 % of women who had cesarean birth [11, 14]. Prevention is the best form of treatment, but the knowledge of pelvic floor changes occurring during pregnancy and delivery is still limited. Complete and accurate understanding of injury mechanisms to

G. Ettore • G. Torrisi (✉) • S. Ferraro
Women and Children's Department, Unit of Gynecology and Obstetrics,
ARNAS "Garibaldi-Nesima", Via Palermo 636, Catania, Sicilia 95128, Italy
e-mail: giuseppe.ettore@gmail.com; gabriellatorrisi@tiscali.it

D. Riva, G. Minini (eds.), *Childbirth-Related Pelvic Floor Dysfunction: Risk Factors, Prevention, Evaluation, and Treatment*,
DOI 10.1007/978-3-319-18197-4_10

pelvic floor is essential to plan appropriate strategies of prevention and treatment. However, modern perineal care aims to identify risk factors of pelvic floor damage and minimize mistakes, with both short-term (reduction perineal trauma) and long-term goals (PFD prevention). Several aspects are considered: information, identification of patients at risk, prevention and treatment procedures to be applied during all reproductive phases. This chapter focuses on the best available practice of perineal care during pregnancy, delivery, and postpartum.

10.2 Perineal Care in Pregnancy

10.2.1 Information and Education

Pregnant women are generally motivated for lifestyle changes and this may be the optimal time to introduce a new behavior. *Life style recommendations* should be addressed to all pregnant women to prevent PFD and it would be useful to develop educational PFD prevention programs based on available evidence.

The following recommendations during pregnancy are prooved to be effective:

- Correct micturition (postures and times)
- Adequate ingestion of fluids
- Perineal hygienic measures
- Intestinal regularity
- Weight control
- Smoking cessation
- Regular examinations of perineal areas
- Encourage women to perform pelvic floor muscular training (PFMT) during pregnancy

Unfortunately during pregnancy, counseling on these issues occurs less frequently than education on general topics like high blood pressure, weight control, diabetes, and pre-eclampsia [15]. This reveals a great potential for the pelvic floor education in daily pregnancy care.

10.2.2 Identification of Antenatal Risk Factors

The antenatal identification of *risk factors* for PFD should be considered in routine obstetrical activity and should become an integral part of the perineal care. The challenge for practitioners is to identify *high-risk* groups and implement preventive practices avoiding unnecessary interventions. It is feasible to give information about antenatal perineal prevention program to all pregnant women, but it is very difficult for logistic and economic reasons to implement the training pelvic program to all pregnant women.

In agreement with other studies [16–23] our experience [11] identifies the following antenatal risk factors:

- Maternal age >35 years
- Family history of urinary or anal incontinence
- Antenatal BMI >30
- Chronic cough
- Constipation
- New onset of UI or AI during pregnancy

The latter represents one of the most important risk factors for persisting postnatal symptoms [11, 21–23].

10.2.3 Methods Proposed to Prevent/Reduce the Genital Tract Trauma and the PFD Developing

10.2.3.1 Antenatal Perineal Massage

All women undergo stretching of pelvic floor during birth, but only some of them experience perineal injury. Genetic predisposition and individual anatomical features such as viscoelastic properties of the vaginal wall, the pubovisceral muscle, and the perineal body are likely to play a role in this process. Studies performed in pregnant rodents [24, 25] show that hormones affect the biochemical composition of solid matrix and water content of each tissue layer of pelvic floor. Remodeling mechanisms lead to changes within the organization, orientation, and diameter of the collagen fibers as well as the crimp structure of the collagen fibrils. Such effects can significantly affect the short- and the long-term viscoelastic properties of vaginal wall, pubovisceral muscles, and perineal body. These data support the use of the *perineal massage* during the last month of pregnancy as a procedure to increase flexibility of the perineal muscles and, therefore, decrease muscular resistance, enabling the perineum to stretch at delivery without tearing or needing episiotomy.

The effect of perineal massage during pregnancy has been evaluated in a few trials. The two major randomized trials were carried out in United Kingdom [26] and Canada [27] with opposite conclusions. However, a Cochrane review in 2013 [28] including four trials (2,497 women) showed that perineal massage, undertaken by the woman or her partner (for as little as once or twice a week starting from the 35th week), reduced the likelihood of perineal trauma, the need for episiotomy (16 % reduction), and subsequent perineal pain. The impact was more evident for nulliparous women than for multiparous women. No significant differences were observed in the incidence of instrumental deliveries, sexual satisfaction, or incontinence of urine, feces or flatus for any women who practiced perineal massage compared to those who did not. Women reported that in the first few weeks massage can be uncomfortable, unpleasant and even produce a painful or burning sensation. However, pain and burning sensation decreased or subsided by the second or third week of massage. Although there is some transient discomfort, perineal massage is generally well accepted by women.

10.2.4 Antenatal Pelvic Floor Muscle Training

Pelvic floor muscle training (PFMT) was proposed for prevention of long-term maternal morbidity (urinary and fecal incontinence) in antenatal women. A Cochrane Review [29] showed that even women who did not leak during pregnancy could reduce the chance of leaking in the first 6 months after childbirth by doing the exercises during and after their pregnancy. The exercises may especially be helpful for primiparous who are at higher risk of suffering urine leakage. During the training the women learn how to perform the so-called *slow or isometric Kegel exercises* and the *isotonic or fast Kegel* exercises with the goal of becoming aware about the correct use of its perineal structure. An example of an effective protocol to treat and prevent urinary incontinence was proposed by Mørkved [30]. Pregnant women are guided by a skilled physiotherapist and each session lasts 45–60 min. The PFMT is performed in lying, sitting, kneeling (Fig. 10.1), and standing positions with legs apart. The physiotherapist encourages the women to perform PFM contractions close to the maximal effort, and to hold the contraction 6–8 s. At the end of each contraction, the women are asked to add 3–4 fast contractions. The resting period is about 6 s. In addition, the women performed 2–3 sets of 10 equally intensive PFM contractions per day at home. The training period in pregnant women was 12 weeks. However, this beneficial effect did not continue on the long-term [31, 32] and novel interventions [33] may be required to improve motivation and adherence for better long-term outcomes. The efficacy of a training program is highly dependent on the patient's adherence and the physiotherapist plays a pivotal role in motivating the patient to follow the pelvic floor muscle (PFM) training protocol.

In conclusion, continent pregnant women having their first baby should be offered a supervised and intensive antepartum PFMT program to prevent postpartum UI/AI (Grade A of Recommendation) and the usual or standard approach

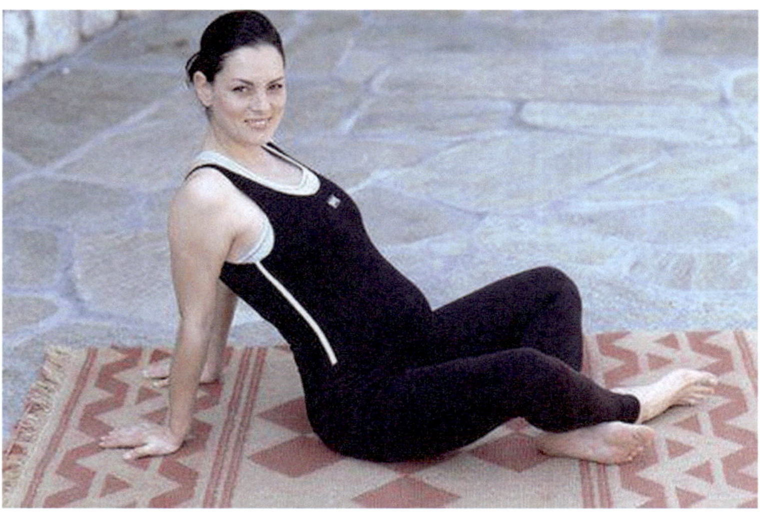

Fig. 10.1 PMFT in pregnancy

to PFMT in pregnancy (which is commonly verbal or written instruction without confirmation of correct contraction or supervision of training) needs to be reviewed.

10.3 Perineal Care in Delivery

About 85 % of women ungergo some degree of perineal trauma during vaginal childbirth. The accurate assessment, recognition and treatment of pelvic floor trauma have gained increasing importance over the last decade and any method proven to reduce the likelihood of sustained genital tract trauma should be recommended. *Perineal trauma* can occur spontaneously or result from a surgical incision of the perineum. Anterior perineal trauma is an injury to the labia, anterior vagina, urethra, or clitoris, and is usually associated with little morbidity. Posterior perineal trauma represents any injury to the posterior vaginal wall, perineal muscles, or anal sphincter. Superficial perineal trauma may be associated with deeper injuries involving structural components of *pelvic floor*, especially *levator ani* (LA) *muscle*.

Using MRI and 3D ultrasound (Figs. 10.2 and 10.3) it is now possible to identify *obstetrical injuries* to LA muscle, particularly to the puborectalis muscle [33–35]. LA muscle trauma has been found in 15–35 % of vaginally parous women [33] and has been shown to be a strong risk factor for PFD later in life [36].

Perineal care in the *second stage of labor* often follows tradition-based routines rather than evidence-based practices. An appropriate management requires the identification of the numerous factors which are potential determinants of severe perineal trauma – nulliparity, a large baby, prolonged second stage and malposition, episiotomy and instrumental delivery [37, 38] – and consequently the evaluation of benefits and risks of different interventions aimed to assist women during pushing.

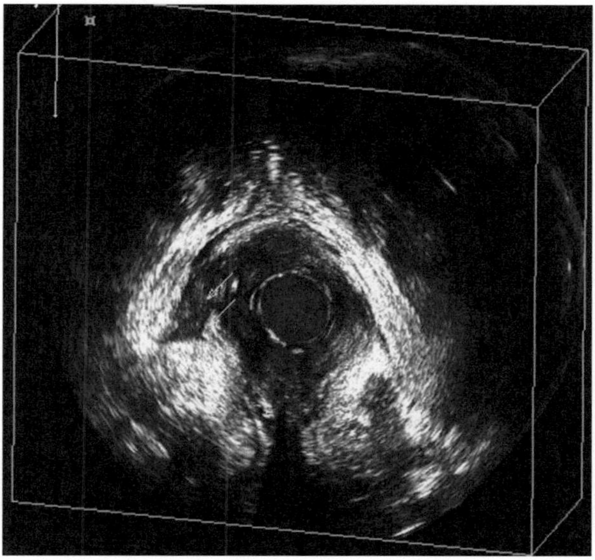

Fig. 10.2 Bilateral levator ani injury in postpartum. (*yellow arrows* point to the right-side injury)

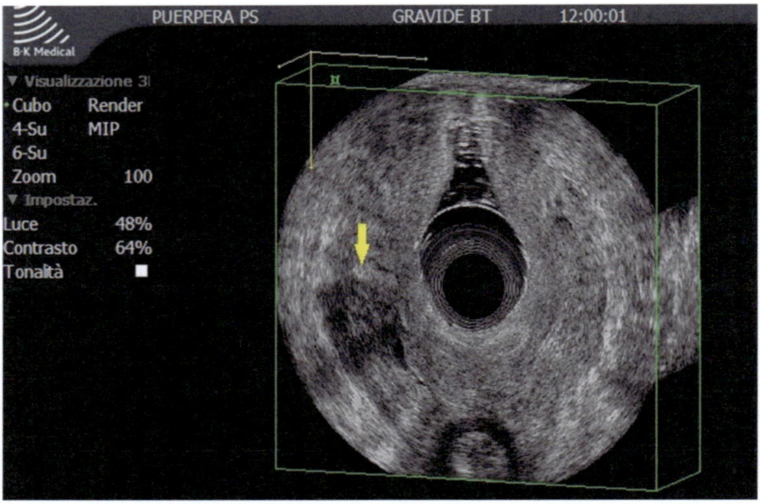

Fig. 10.3 Unilateral levator ani injury (indicated by *yellow arrow*) in postpartum

Obstetric practice underwent major changes during the last few decades, such as a significant increase caesarean section rate, reduction of forceps use, selective use of episiotomy, a preference for mediolateral episiotomy, and delivery in older age. Hence *perineal care* has changed in order to adapt to the new needs. In this chapter, we intend to review the literature on the evidence-based interventions used during the second stage of labor, including maternal position changes, delayed pushing, directed or coached pushing, water delivery, epidural analgesia and perineal techniques for preventing perineal trauma, to update the knowledge and the practice of optimal perineal care.

10.3.1 Perineal Techniques and Other Interventions During the Second Stage of Labor for Reducing Perineal Trauma

Different techniques and interventions are used and some of them were proven beneficial in randomized controlled trials, but others are still lacking evidence of effectiveness.

10.3.2 Interventions with Evidence from Randomized Controlled Trials

10.3.2.1 The Perineal Management Techniques

The Perineal management techniques (flexion technique "Hands-on Approach" and *Ritgen's maneuver*) are the most widely used and are claimed to reduce perineal trauma by reducing the presenting diameter of the fetal head through the woman's vaginal opening and slowing down the birth of the head so to allow the perineum to stretch slowly. The flexion technique involves the maintenance of flexion of fetal head, by exerting pressure on the emerging occiput in a downward direction,

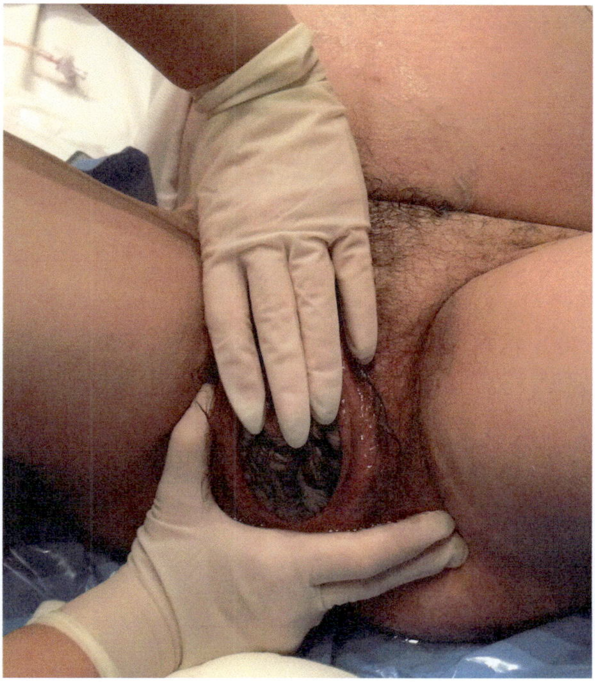

Fig. 10.4 "Hands-on" technique

preventing its extension until crowning, and placing a hand against the perineum to support this structure.

In Ritgen's maneuver, the fetal chin is reached in an area between the anus and coccyx and pulled interiorly, while using the finger of the other hand on the fetal occiput to control delivery speed and keep the fetal head flexed [39]. The Ritgen's maneuver is called modified [40] when performed during a contraction, rather than between contractions as originally recommended.

The "Hands-off Approach" *is a* well documented [41] *birth technique*: the accoucheur has his/her hands poised to readily touch the head of the baby and guard the perineum when necessary (if rapid expulsion of the head is occurring then the accoucheur will be able to apply light pressure to the head), allowing the shoulders to birth spontaneously. The National Institute for Health and Clinical Excellence (NICE) Intrapartum Care Guideline 2007 [42], states that both birth techniques are appropriate to facilitate spontaneous vaginal delivery. A Cochrane review [43] carried out a meta-analysis of 8 RCTs (involving more than 11,000 women) regarding the perineal management techniques and concluded that: "Hands off (or poised)" and "Hands on" showed no significant difference in frequency of intact perineum, laceration rates and third- and fourth-degree tears, but "hands off" is more effective in reducing the rate of episiotomy.

No significant differences in the risk of severe perineal trauma and episiotomy were observed when comparing modified Ritgen's maneuver versus standard techniques.

National Plan Programme in Norway to reduce obstetric anal sphincter injury (OASIS) rate employing a "hands-on technique" (Fig. 10.4) also showed a significant reduction in the incidence of obstetric anal sphincter tears from 4–5 % to 1–2 % during the study period ($P < .001$). LEVEL OF EVIDENCE II [44, 45].

Fig. 10.5 Application of the thumb and index finger to the surface of the perineum

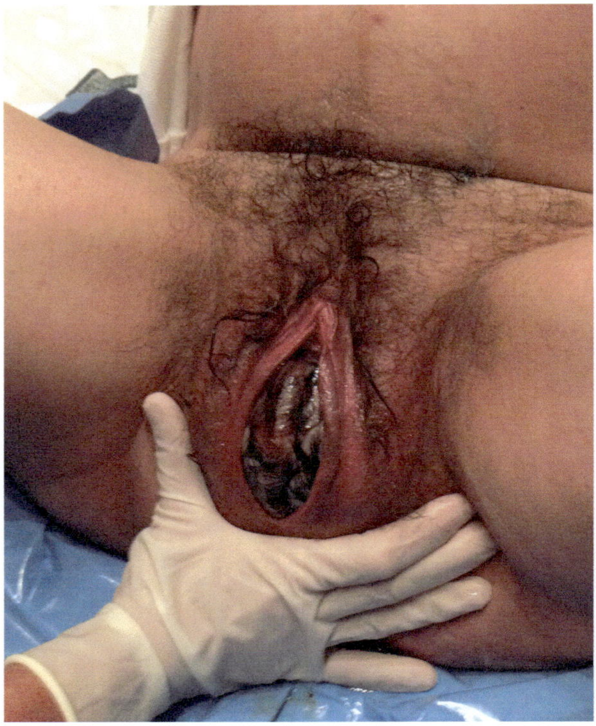

The above perineum protection program consisted of four components during the last part of the second stage of delivery (when the baby's head is crowning):

- Manually slowing down the delivery of the fetal head
- Supporting/protecting perineum with the other hand and squeezing with fingers (first and second) from the perineum lateral parts towards the middle in order to lower the pressure in middle posterior perineum
- Instructing to the delivering woman not to push
- Correcting the quality of episiotomy technique

This perineum protection programme (PEERS 5P's Project) is supported by the results of biomechanical assessment with a finite element model of vaginal delivery, where the appropriate application of the thumb and index finger of the accoucheur's hand to the surface of the perineum (Fig. 10.5) significantly reduces tissue tension throughout the entire thickness of the perineum [46].

10.3.2.2 Position in the Second Stage of Labor

In primitive cultures, women naturally give birth in upright positions like kneeling, standing, or squatting (Fig. 10.6). In western societies, doctors have influenced women to give birth on their backs, sometimes with their legs up in stirrups.

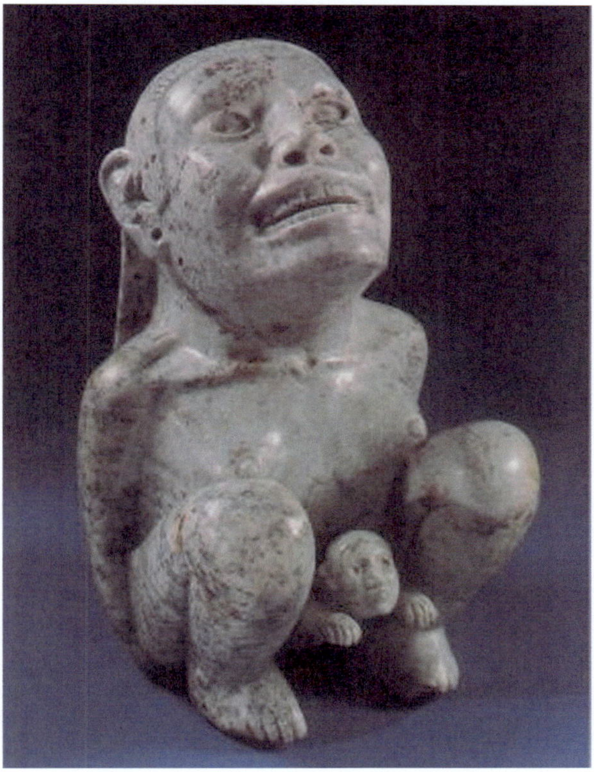

Fig. 10.6 Goddess of fertility in the act of giving birth

The upright positions favor:

- The descent of fetus exploiting the force of gravity
- The increase of pelvis diameter fostering better engagement of the fetus through the birth canal (with particular reference to squatting and kneeling position)
- The reduction of risk of compression of the blood vessels (aorta and cava), and therefore of fetus oxygenation
- The induction of more effective and intense uterine contractions with longer pause between contractions
- The reduced need for medical procedures such as episiotomy and Kristeller maneuver

An Australian retrospective analysis of 2002 [47] evaluated the effects of 6 different *birth positions* on perineal outcomes including episiotomy, lacerations requiring suture, and intact perineum. The authors found that the lateral birth position had the highest rate of intact perineum (66.6 % intact, 28.3 % lacerations requiring suture), whereas squatting was associated with the highest rate of lacerations (41.9 % intact perineum, 53.2 % lacerations requiring suture).

The Cochrane review [48] analyzed 22 studies involving 7,280 women and found that non-supine positions were associated with less assisted births, episiotomies, and fetal heart rate abnormalities, but with more second-degree lacerations. Furthermore, there are no conclusive data about the effect of position for the second stage of labor for women with epidural analgesia and therefore women with epidural analgesia should be encouraged to use whatever position they find comfortable in the second stage of labor.

In summary, there is good evidence that supine positioning should be avoided in second-stage labor. Squatting or sitting may be of benefit when second stage is prolonged or expeditious birth is indicated, while side-lying or hands–knees positions may help prevent lacerations. Therefore, women should be discouraged from lying supine or semi-supine in the second stage of labor and should be encouraged to adopt any other position that they find most comfortable [49].

10.3.2.3 Pushing in the Second Stage of Labor

Interventions during the passive and active phases of the second stage of labor have also been considered to reduce perineal trauma.

- *Delayed pushing* is theorized to promote passive fetal descent and rotation, decrease maternal fatigue, and increase the rate of spontaneous vaginal birth [50]. Indeed, most midwives (85 %) report that *delayed pushing* is their typical practice for women with epidural analgesia [51]. The evidence supporting delayed pushing with epidural analgesia is also fairly robust. Delayed pushing may result in a longer second stage, but it is associated with an increase in the rate of unassisted vaginal births [52, 53], and decreased perineal trauma [54]. The Pushing Early or Pushing Late with Epidurals (PEOPLE) study [52] indicates that delayed pushing when the fetus is occipito posterior (OP) may increase the chance for spontaneous vaginal birth without the need for rotational or instrumental intervention.
- *Directed versus spontaneous pushing*. Research evidence does not support the use of *directed pushing*. Bloom et al. [55] conducted a trial of coached and uncoached pushing in the second stage of labor. The duration of the second stage of labor is shorter with coached pushing (mean difference 18.59 min), but no statistical difference was identified in the number of instrumental/operative deliveries, perineal tears, postpartum hemorrhage, neonatal outcomes. In addition, urodynamic factors measured 3 months postpartum were negatively affected by directed pushing. Measures of first urge to void and bladder capacity were decreased (mean difference respectively 41.50 ml, 95 % CI 8.40–74.60, and 54.60 ml, 95 % CI 13.31–95.89) [56].

10.3.2.4 Duration of Second Stage

The average duration of both first and second stages of labor have trended up in the recent decades, and it is postulated that increased rates of epidural analgesia use and other maternal demographics are at least partly responsible [38, 51, 55]. There is a strong association between *prolonged second stage* and increased maternal morbidity: large retrospective and prospective observational studies report increased rates of third- and fourth-degree lacerations [25, 26] and other maternal complication – uterine atony, postpartum hemorrhage, intrapartum fever, and hysterectomy [47]– following prolonged second stage or pushing for more than 3 h or 4 h. The American College of Obstetrics and Gynecology (ACOG) hence recommends considering the diagnosis of prolonged second stage in nulliparous woman after 3 h with regional anesthesia or 2 h without, and for multiparous women after 2 h with regional anesthesia or 1 h without [57].

In conclusion:

- The routine use of Valsalva pushing in the second stage of labor is not helpful.
- Delayed pushing for women with epidural analgesia, especially when the fetal station is high or fetal position is not anterior, increases the chance of having a spontaneous vaginal birth.
- Directing women on when and how to push should be considered an intervention to be used only when indicated because spontaneous pushing is usually safer for the mother and fetus.
- Each woman should be individually assessed and instructed on the potential risks to her and the fetus of a prolonged second stage of labor.

10.3.2.5 Water Immersion in Labor and Birth

Evidence suggests that *water immersion* during the first stage of labor reduces the perception of pain [41], the use of epidural/spinal analgesia, and the duration of the first stage of labor [58]. Furthermore, several studies have shown that delivery in water reduce the frequency and severity of perineal injuries, because immersion in hot water promotes relaxation of perineum tissues [59, 60]. On the contrary, Cochrane review [58] and our data [61] could not find significant differences between usual delivery and water delivery regarding rate of episiotomy, second-, third-, and fourth-degree tears.

10.3.2.6 Warm Compresses

A recently published meta-analysis [43], assessing the effect of holding *warm gauzes* against the perineum, showed that such procedure is more effective than hands off or no warm compression in preventing the incidence of third- and fourth-degree tears and concluded that there is sufficient evidence to support the use of warm compresses in the second stage of labor.

In addition, treated women reported significantly lower pain score after birth and this simple and inexpensive procedure has been shown to be acceptable to both women and midwives.

10.3.2.7 Perineal Massage During the Second Stage of Labor

The stretching massage of the perineum during each contraction is used to ease the perineum back over the head as it crowns. Two studies [62, 63] comparing massage versus "hands off" or usual care showed that the risk of third- and fourth-degree tears was significantly lower in the massage group, but the intervention did not increase the likelihood of an intact perineum and nor reduce the risk of pain and dyspareunia. Therefore, according to NICE guidance [41] perineal massage should not be performed in the second stage of labor.

10.3.2.8 Episiotomy

Episiotomy is the topic of another chapter of this book. However, regarding to perineal trauma prevention, the recent review of Hunter [64] showed that restrictive use of episiotomy appears to give a reduced number of side effects compared with routine episiotomy. Women experienced less severe perineal trauma, especially posterior perineal trauma, less suturing, but no difference in occurrence of pain, urinary or anal incontinence, and painful sex. Episiotomy should be performed if there is a clinical indication such as instrumental birth or suspected fetal compromise.

10.3.2.9 Instrumental Delivery

Perineal trauma is more likely to occur with *forceps delivery*, therefore, the Royal College of Obstetricians and Gynaecologists recommends that the vacuum extractor should be the instrument of choice for operative vaginal birth [65].

10.3.2.10 Epidural Analgesia in Labor

Epidural has become an increasingly popular method of pain relief for women in labor. Evidence suggests that epidural or combined spinal-epidural (CSE) does effectively manage pain in labor, but may increase the rate of adverse effects. A Cochrane review on epidural versus non-epidural or no analgesia in labor [66], including 38 randomized controlled studies and involving 9,658 women, showed that *epidural analgesia* was associated with an increased risk of assisted vaginal birth, sutured perineal trauma, longer second stage of labor, and urinary retention. During pregnancy, women should be told about the benefits and potential adverse effects on themselves and their babies of the different methods of pain control and they should be let free to choose whatever pain management during labor.

10.3.2.11 Continuous Support During Labor

There is some evidence of benefit of continuous one-to-one intrapartum support from a midwife compared with usual care, in terms of reducing the rate of instrumental deliveries. However, the overall rates of perineal trauma were not reduced [1].

10.3.3 Techniques to Reduce Perineal Trauma with Weaker Evidence

10.3.3.1 Antenatal Pelvic Floor Muscle Training

Pelvic floor muscle training (PFMT) is commonly recommended both during pregnancy and after the birth to prevent and treat incontinence [29], but the effect on perineal trauma is not known yet. In a large cohort study [67] PFMT in pregnancy was not associated with increased risk of perineal trauma.

10.3.3.2 Manual Rotation of the Fetal Head

During the first stage of labor, 10–34 % of fetuses are in *occipito-posterior (OP) position*. Persistent OP can result in a longer second stage and is associated with an increased risk for surgical or instrumental birth [68] and severe perineal tears. Therefore, it is important to accurately diagnose fetal position and utilize interventions that encourage rotation to OA position. Usual care in the case of OP position is to wait spontaneous rotation to OA position. Manual rotation of the fetal head from OP to OA has been shown to be a successful intervention and can reduce the incidence of cesarean and vacuum-assisted births [69]. Evidence from the PEOPLE study suggests that delayed pushing when the fetus is OP may increase the chance for spontaneous vaginal birth without the need for rotational or instrumental intervention [52]. Specific maternal positions, such as kneeling on "hands and knees," could facilitate the rotation from OP to OA position. World Health Organization encourages walking and changing of maternal position to promote spontaneous rotation of the fetal head in OA position during labor [70]. A Cochrane review [71] on the effects of "hands and knees" posture on fetal malposition (lateral or posterior) concluded that the adoption of this posture 10 min daily in late pregnancy has the short-term potential to change the fetal position and reduce lumbar pain, and that its use in labor was associated with reduced backache, but did not influence delivery outcomes and could be recommended as an intervention.

10.4 Care and Assessment of Woman Immediately Following Birth

Systematic inspection of genital area is recommended to assess the extent of perineal trauma and structures involved. In addition, rectal examination should also be performed to evaluate whether any damage occurred to the external or internal anal sphincter.

The following basic principles should be observed when performing perineal repair [41]:

- *Severe trauma* should be repaired by an experienced practitioner under regional or general anesthesia. An indwelling catheter should be inserted for 24 h to prevent urinary retention.
- Good anatomical alignment of the wound should be achieved and consideration given to the cosmetic results.
- Information should be given to the woman regarding the extent of the trauma, the method of repair, and the importance of pelvic-floor exercises for functional rehabilitation

10.4.1 Suturing Methods and Materials

Relevant factors in the reduction of perineal trauma are suturing methods and materials. Traditionally, the vagina is stitched using a continuous locking stitch and the perineal muscles and skin are repaired using approximately three or four individual stitches, each needing to be knotted separately to prevent them from dislodging. For more than 70 years the "continuous non-locking stitching method" has been preferred to "traditional interrupted methods." A Cochrane systematic review [72] based on data from 16 randomized controlled trials involving 8,184 women, showed that continuous versus interrupted *suturing techniques* for perineal closure are associated with less short-term pain, need for analgesia and suture removal. Rapidly absorbable synthetic sutures are less likely to be associated with the need to remove suture materials and rapidly absorbable polyglactin suture (Vicryl Rapide W) is the material of choice. Indeed, the NICE intrapartum guidelines [41] recommend the combined use of continuous suturing and rapidly absorbable synthetic materials.

Two particular conditions of perineal care in labor are those dealing with women with a history of *severe perineal trauma* or with infibulated genital mutilation.

Women with a history of severe perineal trauma should be informed that their risk of repeat severe perineal trauma is not increased in a subsequent birth, compared with women having their first baby. However, to make an informed choice on the future mode of birth, the following issues should to be discussed:

- Current urgency or incontinence symptoms
- The degree of previous trauma
- The risk of recurrence
- The success of previous repair
- The psychological effect of the previous trauma

Women with *infibulated genital mutilation* should be informed on the risks of delay in the second stage and spontaneous laceration together with the need for an anterior episiotomy or defibulation in labor.

10.5 Perineal Care in Postpartum

Care and assessment of the woman immediately after birth includes both physical and psychological issues and the perineal care is only one aspect of routine *postnatal care* for women and their babies. The woman should be fully involved in planning the timing and the content of each postnatal care consultation.

Good communication between health care professionals and the woman is essential. It should be supported by provision of evidence-based information offered in a form that is tailored to the needs of the individual woman and the woman's cultural practices should be taken into account. A distinction should be made between short-term postpartum perineal care and long-term perineal care which is of course a more articulated and complex condition.

10.5.1 Short-Term Postpartum Care

Women should be advised about the importance of *perineal hygiene*, including frequent changing of sanitary pads, washing hands before and after doing it, and daily bathing or showering to keep their perineum clean. A special attention should be given to recovery of urinary and fecal functionality. If spontaneous *micturition* is

Fig. 10.7 "Postpartum" card

WOMEN AND CHILDREN'S DEPARTMENT
UNIT OF GYNECOLOGY AND OBSTETRICS
Chairman: Prof. Giuseppe Ettore
"GARIBALDI-NESIMA" Hospital Catania
Pelvic floor dysfunctions Post-partum card

Surname ____________ Name ___________
age _________ Telephone _________

BMI ☐ Panity ☐ Constipation: yes ☐ no ☐
UI positive family history:
Genital prolapse positive family history: yes ☐ no ☐
AI positive family history: yes ☐ no ☐

Delivery: PS ☐ PO ☐ CS ☐
Intact perineum: yes ☐ no ☐
Perineal tears 1° ☐ 2° ☐ 3° ☐ 4° ☐
UI onset: in pregnancy ☐ post-partum ☐
AI onset: in pregnancy ☐ post-partum ☐

not achieved by 6 h after birth and measures to encourage micturition are not immediately successful, bladder volume should be assessed and catheterization considered. Women who are constipated should have their diet and fluid intake assessed and a gentle laxative may be recommended if dietary measures are not effective. Women with hemorrhoids should be advised to take dietary measures to avoid constipation and should be offered management based on local treatment protocols. Early *postpartum* period is a valuable time for the prevention of PFD.

We suggest that before discharging a patient, a form should be filled out for each puerpera reporting every risk factor (personal or obstetric), like the one in Fig. 10.7. We believe that *screening* in postpartum is an important step because it allows to identify women still asymptomatic, but susceptible of developing PFD.

At each postnatal visit the health care professional should assess the perineum if the woman complains about abnormalities of perineal healing process, including perineal pain, discomfort or stinging, offensive smell or dyspareunia. Women should be advised that topical cold therapy, for example, crushed ice or gel pads, are effective methods for perineal pain relief. If oral analgesia is required, paracetamol should be the drug of choice unless contraindicated. If cold therapy or paracetamol are not effective, a prescription for oral or rectal non-steroidal anti-inflammatory (NSAID) medication may be considered. Women should be asked about resumption of *sexual activity* and possible dyspareunia 2–6 weeks after the birth. A water-based lubricant gel may be advised to help ease discomfort during intercourse, particularly if a woman is breastfeeding [73].

10.5.2 Long-Term Perineal Care

The first evaluation for patients who had an eventful *puerperium* may be scheduled at 6 weeks and must include a complete medical history, physical examination and a careful assessment of the perineum with 2D *transperineal ultrasound* for the evaluation of urethral hypermobility and 3D transperineal or *transvaginal ultrasound* for the assessment of *urogenital hiatus* area and LA avulsion [33–35]. The main goals of this first evaluation are prevention and treatment of symptomatic patients.

Prevention High-risk patients (e.g., obese women or those with antenatal UI/AI, large babies, forceps delivery, LA avulsion, increased bladder neck mobility) [35, 74] shall be offered rehabilitation programs which is currently the only valid instrument to lower the development of PFD symptoms.

Treatment Women with urinary or fecal incontinence should be assessed for severity, duration, and frequency of symptoms and treated with appropriate interventions.

PFMT in postnatal women is the adequate therapy in case of persistent postpartum urinary or anal incontinence and the recovery of a fully functional perineal structure requires the involvement of supplementary muscle-dependent mechanisms.

The training involves exercises that women ought to do several times a day to strengthen their pelvic floor muscles. They are usually taught by a health professional such as a physiotherapist. The *kinesitherapy* must be performed no later than 6 weeks from delivery. It includes at least 12 sessions conducted by the same operator and in an appropriate environment. Fundamental is also the enhancement of patient compliance to home training.

A recent Cochrane review about the outcomes of PFMT [75] in 8,485 women (4,231 PFMT, 4,254 controls) with persistent UI 3 months after delivery concluded that patients receiving PFMT showed a 40 % reduction of UI at 12 months compared to untreated patients.

Furthermore, women receiving PFMT after delivery exhibited an overall 50 % decrease in fecal incontinence compared the control group.

The treatment reveals more effective when the intervention is intensive.

However, there is not enough evidence to suggest that these effects last beyond the first year.

The efficacy of a training program is highly dependent on the women's the adherence to the program. Poor adherence to pelvic floor exercise regimens can act as an additional barrier to health professional intervention. In prevention and treatment one important part of the physiotherapist's role is to motivate the patient to follow the pelvic floor muscle (PFM) training protocol. The acceptability of a training program also depends on the simplicity and time needed to perform the exercises.

Conclusions

This chapter reviewed perineal care interventions that may help to minimize perineal trauma. Preventing the *childbirth trauma* is likely to benefit large numbers of women and it may also result in cost savings and improvement in quality of life. Defining the best approach for perineal care during pregnancy, delivery, and postpartum and to identify women who could benefit from a specific diagnostic, prophylactic, and therapeutic program to prevent and treat long-term consequences is a complex task. Based on available evidence this goal could be achieved only through a stepwise model: first, by tailored counseling on the basis of patient's characteristics, obstetric history, and evaluation of *pelvic dysfunctions* already present before and during pregnancy; secondly, by careful management of second stage of labor; thirdly, through a systematic search for PFD during scheduled postpartum examinations. Thus health services for pregnant and postpartum women should include strategies to prevent and treat PFD, but presently most health care systems do not provide adequate care to these issues. Collaboration among gynecologists, midwifes, and physiotherapists ensures consistency across health professionals dealing with pregnant women and is mandatory to reach a high quality of care.

References

1. Kettle C, Tohill S (2008) Perineal care. Clinical Evidence. http://www.ncbi.nlm.nih.gov/pubmed/19445799. Accessed 20 June 2012
2. Ashton-Miller JA, DeLanceyJ OL (2009) On the biomechanics of vaginal birth and common sequelae. Annu Rev Biomed Eng 11:163–176
3. Memon H, Handa VL (2012) Pelvic floor disorders following vaginal or cesarean delivery. Curr Opin Obstet Gynecol 24:349–354. doi:10.1097/GCO.0b013e328357628b
4. Albers L, Garcia J, Renfrew M, McCandlish R, Elbourne D (1999) Distribution of genital tract trauma in childbirth and related postnatal pain. Birth 26(1):11–17
5. Glazener CM, Abdalla M, Stroud P, Naji S, Templeton A, Russell IT (1995) Postnatal maternal morbidity: extent, causes, prevention and treatment. Br J Obstet Gynaecol 102(4):282–287
6. McCandlish R, Bowler U, van Asten H, Berridge G, Winter C, Sames L, Garcia J, Renfrew M, Elbourne D (1998) A randomised controlled trial of care of the perineum during second stage of normal labour. Br J Obstet Gynaecol 105(12):1262–1272
7. Barret G, Pendry E, Peacock J, Victor C, Thakar R, Manyonda I (2000) Women's sexual health after childbirth. Br J Obstet Gynaecol 107:186–195
8. Andrews V, Thakar R, Sultan AH, Jones PW (2007) Evaluation of postpartum perineal pain and dyspareunia – a prospective study. Eur J Obstet Gynecol Reprod Biol 137:152–156
9. Glazener CM, Herbison GP, MacArthur C, Lancashire R, McGee MA, Grant AM, Wilson PD (2006) New postnatal urinary incontinence: obstetric and other risk factors in primiparae. BJOG 113:208–217
10. Hansen BB, Svare J, Viktrup L, Jørgensen T, Lose G (2012) Urinary incontinence during pregnancy and 1 year after delivery in primiparous women compared with a control group of nulliparous women. Neurourol Urodyn 31:475–480
11. Torrisi G, Minini G, Bernasconi F, Perrone A, Trezza G, Guardabasso V, Ettore G (2012) A prospective study of pelvic floor dysfunctions related to delivery. Eur J Obstet Gynecol Reprod Biol 160:110–115
12. Eason E, Labrecque M, Marcoux S, Mondor M (2002) Anal incontinence after childbirth. Can Med Assoc J 166(3):326–330
13. Raisanen S, Vehvilainen-Julkunen K, Gissler M, Heinonen S (2011) High episiotomy rate protects from obstetric anal sphincter ruptures: a birth register-study on delivery intervention policies in Finland. Scand J Public Health 39:457–463
14. Diez-Itza I, Arrue M, Ibanez L (2011) Influence of mode of delivery on pelvic organ support 6 months postpartum. Gynecol Obstet Invest 72:123–129
15. McLennan MT, Melick CF, Alten B, Young J, Hoehn MR (2006) Patients' knowledge of potentiale pelvic floor changes associated with pregnancy and delivery. Int Urogynecol J Pelvic Floor Dysfunct 17(1):22–26

16. Dietz-Itza I, Arrue M, Ibanez L, Murgiondo A, Paredes J, Sarasqueta C (2010) Factors involved in stress urinary incontinence 1 year after first delivery. Int Urogynecol J 21:439–445
17. Gyhagen M, Bullarbo M, Nielsen TF, Milsom I (2013) Prevalence and risk factors for pelvic organ prolapse 20 years after childbirth: a national cohort study in singleton primiparae after vaginal or caesarean delivery. BJOG 120(2):152–160
18. Hijaz A, Sadeghi Z, Byrne L, Hou JC, Daneshgari F (2012) Advanced maternal age as a risk factor for stress urinary incontinence: a review of the literature. Int Urogynecol J 23:395–401. doi:10.1007/s00192-011-1562-5
19. Zhu L, Li L, Lang JH, Xu T (2012) Prevalence and risk factors for peri- and postpartum urinary incontinence in primiparous women in China: a prospective longitudinal study. Int Urogynecol J 23:563–572. doi:10.1007/s00192-011-1640-8
20. Gartland D, Donath S, MacArthur C, Brown SJ (2012) The onset, recurrence and associated obstetric risk factors for urinary incontinence in the first 18 months after a first birth: an Australian nulliparous cohort study. BJOG 119(11):1361–1369
21. Martin-Martin S, Pascual-Fernandez A, Alvarez-Colomo C, Calvo-Gonzalez R, Muñoz-Moreno M, Cortiñas-Gonzalez JR, Sangsawang BJR (2014) Urinary incontinence during pregnancy and postpartum. Associated risk factors and influence of pelvic floor exercises. Arch Esp Urol 67(4):323–330
22. Sangsawang B (2014) Risk factors for the development of stress urinary incontinence during pregnancy in primigravidae: a review of the literature. Eur J Obstet Gynecol Reprod Biol. doi:10.1016/j.ejogrb.2014.04.010
23. Liang CC, Wu MP, Lin SJ, Lin YJ, Chang SD, Wang HH (2013) Clinical impact of and contributing factors to urinary incontinence in women 5 years after first delivery. Int Urogynecol J 24:99–104. doi:10.1007/s00192-012-1855-3
24. Rahn DD, Ruff MD, Brown SA (2008) Biomechanical properties of the vaginal wall: effect of pregnancy, elastic fiber deficiency, and pelvic organ prolapse. Am J Obstet Gynecol 198:590
25. Zong W, Jallah ZC, Stein SE (2010) Repetitive mechanical stretch increases extracellular collagenase activity in vaginal fibroblasts. Female Pelvic Med Reconstr Surg 16:257–262
26. Shipman MK, Boniface DR, Tefft ME, McCloghry F (1997) Antenatal perineal massage and subsequent perineal outcomes: a randomized controlled trial. Br J Obstet Gynaecol 104:787–791
27. Labreque M, Eason E, Marcoux S (1999) Randomized trial of perineal massage during pregnancy. Am J Obstet Gynecol 180:593–600
28. Beckmann MM, Stock OM (2013) Antenatal perineal massage for reducing perineal trauma Cochrane Database Syst Rev. doi:10.1002/14651858. CD005123.pub 3
29. Boyle R, Hay-Smith EJ, Cody JD, Mørkved S (2012) Pelvic floor muscle training for prevention and treatment of urinary and faecal incontinence in antenatal and postnatal women. Cochrane Database Syst Rev. doi:10.1002/14651858. CD007471.pub2.
30. Mørkved S, Bø K, Schei B, Salvesen KA (2003) Pelvic floor muscle training during pregnancy to prevent urinary incontinence: a single-blind randomized controlled trial. Obstet Gynecol 101(2):313–319
31. Agur W, Steggles P, Waterfield M, Freeman R (2008) The long-term effectiveness of antenatal pelvic floor muscle training: eight-year follow up of a randomised controlled trial. Br J Obstet Gynaecol 115:985–990; Bø K, Kvarstein B, Nygaard I (2005) Lower urinary tract symptoms and pelvic floor muscle exercise adherence after 15 years. Obstet Gynecol 105(5 Pt 1):999–1005
32. Albers-Heitner P, Berghmans B, Joore M, Lagro-Janssen T, Severens J, Nieman F, Winkens R (2008) The effects of involving a nurse practitioner in primary care for adult patients with urinary incontinence: the PromoCon study (Promoting Continence). BMC Health Serv Res 8:84. doi:10.1186/1472-6963-8-84
33. Dietz HP, Lanzarone V (2005) Levator trauma after vaginal delivery. Obstet Gynecol 106:707–712
34. Shek K, Dietz H (2010) Intrapartum risk factors for levator trauma. BJOG 117:1485–1492
35. Torrisi G, Fonti I, Ferraro S, Galanti S, Ettore G (2013) Three-dimensional Transvaginal ultrasound of the pelvic floor in pregnancy and three months after delivery: an observational study. Neurol Urodyn 32(S1):54–55

36. DeLancey JO, Morgan DM, Fenner DE, Kearney R, Guire K, Miller JM, Hussain H, Umek W, Hsu Y, Ashton-Miller JA (2007) Comparison of levatorani muscle defects and function in women with and without pelvic organ prolapse. Obstet Gynecol 109:295–302; Majida M, Braekken I, Bø K, Benth J, Engh M (2011) Anterior but not posterior compartment prolapse is associated with levator hiatus area: a three- and four-dimensional transperineal ultrasound study. BJOG 118:329–337. doi:10.1111/j.1471-0528.2010.02784.x
37. Laine K, Skjeldestad FE, Sanda B, Horne H, Spydslaug A, Staff AC (2011) Prevalence and risk factors for anal incontinence after obstetric anal sphincter rupture. Acta Obstet Gynecol Scand 90:319–324
38. Groutz A, Cohen A, Gold R, Hasson J, Wengier A, Lessing JB, Gordon D (2011) Risk factors for severe perineal injury during childbirth: a case-control study of 60 consecutive cases. Colorectal Dis 13:e216–e219. doi:10.1111/j.1463-1318.2011.02620.x
39. Cunningham FG (2008) The Ritgen maneuver: another sacred cow questioned. Obstet Gynecol 112:210–211
40. Jonsson ER, Elfaghi I, Rydhstrom H, Herbst A (2008) Modified Ritgen's maneuver for anal sphincter injury at delivery: a randomized controlled trial. Obstet Gynecol 112:212–217
41. National Institute of Clinical Excellence (NICE) (2007) Intrapartum Care: care of healthy women and their babies. RCOG Press, London
42. SouzaCaroci D, da Costa A, Gonzalez Riesco ML (2006) A comparison of "hands off" versus "hands on" techniques for decreasing perineal lacerations during birth. J Midwifery Womens Health 51(2):106–111
43. Aasheim V, Nilsen AB, Lukasse M, Reinar LM (2011) Perineal techniques during the second stage of labour for reducing perineal trauma. Cochrane Database Syst Rev. doi:10.1002/14651858.CD006672.pub2
44. Hals E, Oian P, Pirhonen T, Gissler M, Hjelle S, Nilsen EB, Severinsen AM, Solsletten C, Hartgill T, Pirhonen J (2010) A multicenter interventional program to reduce the incidence of anal sphincter tears. Obstet Gynecol 116:901–908
45. Laine K, Gissler M, Pirhonen J (2009) Changing incidence of anal sphincter tears in four Nordic countries through the last decades. Eur J Obstet Gynecol Reprod Biol 146:71–75
46. Jansova M, Kalis V, Lobovsky L, Hyncik L, Karbanova J, Rusavy Z (2014) The role of thumb and index finger placement in manual perineal protection. Int Urogynecol J 25:1533–1540. doi:10.1007/s00192-014-2425-7
47. Shorten A, Donsante J, Shorten B (2002) Birth position, accoucheur, and perineal outcomes. Informing women about choices for vaginal birth. Birth 29(1):18–27
48. Gupta JK, Hofmeyr GJ, Shehmar M (2012) Position in the second stage of labour for women without epidural anaesthesia. Cochrane Database Syst Rev. doi:10.1002/14651858
49. The Royal College Of Midwives (RCM) (2012) Evidence based guidelines for midwifery-led care in labour: positions for labour and birth. RCM, London
50. Priddis H, Dahlen H, Schmied V (2012) What are the facilitators, inhibitors, and implications of birth positioning? A review of the literature. Women Birth 25:100–106
51. Osborne K, Hanson L (2011) Directive versus supportive approaches used by midwives when providing care during the second stage of labor. J Midwifery Womens Health 57(1):3–11
52. Fraser WD, Marcoux S, Krauss I, Douglas J, Goulet C, Boulvain M (2000) Multicenter, randomized, controlled trial of delayed pushing for nulliparous women in the second stage of labor with continuous epidural analgesia. The PEOPLE (Pushing Early or Pushing Late with Epidural) Study Group. Am J Obstet Gynecol 182(5):1165–1172
53. Tuuli MG, Frey HA, Odibo AO, Macones GA, Cahill AG (2012) Immediate compared with delayed pushing in the second stage of labor: a systematic review and meta-analysis. Obstet Gynecol 120(3):660–668
54. Simpson KR, James DC (2005) Effects of immediate versus delayed pushing during second-stage labor on fetal well-being: a randomized clinical trial. Nurs Res 54(3):149–157
55. Bloom SL, Casey BM, Schaffer JI, McIntire DD, Leveno KJ (2006) A randomized trial of coached versus uncoached maternal pushing during the second stage of labor. Am J Obstet Gynecol 194(1):10–13

56. Schaffer JI, Bloom SL, Casey BM, McIntire DD, Nihira MA, Leveno KJ (2005) A randomized trial of the effects of coached vs uncoached maternal pushing during the second stage of labor on postpartum pelvic floor structure and function. Am J Obstet Gynecol 192(5):1692–1696
57. Caughey AB, Cahill AG, Guise JM, Rouse DJ (2014) American College of Obstetricians and Gynecologists; Society for Maternal-Fetal Medicine. Obstetric care consensus: safe prevention of the primary cesarean delivery. Am J Obstet Gynecol 210(3):179–193
58. Cluett ER, Burns E (2009) Immersion in water in labour and birth. Cochrane Database Syst Rev. doi:10.1002/14651858.CD000111.pub3
59. Dahlen HG, Dowling H, Tracy M, Schmied V, Tracy S (2013) Maternal and perinatal outcomes amongst low risk women giving birth in water compared to six birth positions on land. A descriptive cross sectional study in a birth centre over 12 years. Midwifery 29(7):759–764
60. Bodner K, Bodner-Adler B, Wierrani F, Mayerhofer K, Fokuser C, Niedemyr A, Gruberger W (2002) Effects of water birth on maternal and neonatal outcomes. Wien Klin Wochenschr 114(10–11):391–395
61. Torrisi G, Ettore G, Fonti I, Ferraro S, Pappalardo E, D'Urso E, Guardabasso G (2010) Water birth and perineal dysfunctions: prospective study. Neurol Urodyn. doi:10.1002/nau
62. Albers LL, Sedler KD, Bedrick EJ, Teaf D, Peralta P (2005) Midwifery care measures in the second stage of labor and reduction of genital tract trauma at birth: a randomized trial. J Midwifery Womens Health 50(5):365–372
63. Stamp G, Kruzins G, Crowther C (2001) Perineal massage in labour and prevention of perineal trauma: randomised controlled trial. BMJ 322(7297):1277–1280
64. Carroli G, Mignini L (2009) Episiotomy for vaginal birth. Cochrane Database Syst Rev. doi:10.1002/14651858. CD000081.pub2
65. American College of Obstetrics and Gynecology (ACOG) (2003) Practice Bulletin Number 49: dystocia and augmentation of labor. Obstet Gynecol 102:1445–1454
66. Anim-Somuah M, Smyth RM, Jones L (2011) Epidural versus non-epidural or no analgesia in labour. Cochrane Database Syst Rev. doi:10.1002/14651858. CD000331.pub3
67. Bø K, Fleten C, Nystad W (2009) Effect of antenatal pelvic floor muscle training on labor and birth. Obstet Gynecol 113(6):1279–1284
68. Schiessl B, Janni W, Jundt K, Rammel G, Peschers U, Kainer F (2005) Obstetrical parameters influencing the duration of the second stage of labor. Eur J Obstet Gynecol Reprod Biol 118(1):17–20
69. Shaffer BL, Cheng YW, Vargas JE, Laros RK Jr, Caughey AB (2006) Manual rotation of the fetal occiput: predictors of success and delivery. Am J Obstet Gynecol 194(5):e7–e9
70. World Health Organization, Department of Reproductive Health and Research (2007) Managing complications in pregnancy and childbirth: a guide for midwives and doctors. WHO, Geneva
71. Hunter S, Hofmeyr GJ, Kulier R (2007) Hands and knees posture in late pregnancy or labour for fetal malposition (lateral or posterior). Cochrane Database Syst Rev. doi:10.1002/14651858. CD001063
72. Kettle C, Dowswell T, Ismail KMK (2012) Continuous and interrupted suturing techniques for repair of episiotomy or second-degree tears. Cochrane Database Syst Rev. doi:10.1002/14651858. CD000947.pub3
73. National Institute of Clinical Excellence (NICE) (2006) Postnatal care. Routine postnatal care of women and their babies. RCOG Press, London
74. Reilly ET, Freeman RM, Waterfield MR, Waterfield AE, Steggles P, Pedlar F (2002) Prevention of postpartum stress incontinence in primigravidae with increased bladder neck mobility: a randomised controlled trial of antenatal pelvic floor exercises. BJOG 109(1):68–76
75. Boyle R, Hay-Smith EJ, Cody JD, Mørkved S (2014) Pelvic floor muscle training for prevention and treatment of urinary and fecal incontinence in antenatal and postnatal women: a short version Cochrane review. Neurourol Urodyn 33:269–276. doi:10.1002/nau.22402

Genital Prolapse and Urinary Incontinence After Childbirth

11

Francesco Marson and Luisella Squintone

11.1 Epidemiology

Pelvic floor damage is a well-recognized consequence after childbirth, and a huge number of studies give interesting data regarding its epidemiology. A recent study of Glazener et al. collected data from 3,763 women 12 years after childbirth and found an objective prolapse in 24 % of women; they reported that a body mass index (BMI) over 25 and age over 25 years at first delivery were associated with worse prolapse symptom score (POP-SS), and that in women over 30 years at their first pregnancy there was a significant association with the onset of prolapse [1]. Analyses about risks factors related with prolapse surgery have been made: Women older than 30 years at first vaginal delivery had an incidence of POP surgery of 13.8 %, while in younger women it was only 6.8 % [2]. Prolapse stage usually changes after delivery: Elenskaia et al. reported that 5 years after childbirth the stage of prolapse worsen after vaginal delivery but not after cesarean [3]. Other older studies reported that 50 % of parous women have some degrees of genital prolapse, with 10–20 % symptomatic [4]. Anyway a precise epidemiology about POP is not easily available, due to lack of a standard evaluation. Samuelsson et al. reported that about 44 % of parous women have some form of POP [5]. It is to notice that clinical prolapse evaluation is different from subjective prolapse perception with symptoms: In a study by Durnea et al. with 202 participants despite the high prevalence of POP on POP-Q examination, only 20 % of participants were symptomatic [6].

F. Marson (✉)
Ospedale Città della Salute e della scienza di Torino, Presidio Molinette, 88, Torino 10126, Italy
e-mail: francescomarson84@gmail.com

L. Squintone
Ospedale Città della Salute e della Scienza di Torino,
Presidio CTO-Maria Adelaide, 88, Torino 10126, Italy

D. Riva, G. Minini (eds.), *Childbirth-Related Pelvic Floor Dysfunction: Risk Factors, Prevention, Evaluation, and Treatment*,
DOI 10.1007/978-3-319-18197-4_11

Like pelvic organ prolapse, urinary incontinence (UI) represents a frequent condition after childbirth, and fear for it is a common reason for maternal demand for cesarean delivery, even if the latter is not free of consequences as regards the pelvic floor. The first year after childbirth seems to be the cut off time for restoring a normal continence, a further recovery being considered difficult after that period [7–9]. Stress urinary incontinence (SUI) seems to be the most prevalent type of UI, with 29.1–40.2 % of prevalence after vaginal delivery and 14.2–25.5 % after cesarean across 1 year [10]. Barbosa et al. after a cross-sectional study involving 220 women, reported a 2 years prevalence of UI following vaginal childbirth and cesarean section of 17 % and 18.9 %, respectively [11]. Other studies, conducted on specific populations, reported similar rates of UI after 1 year [12, 13]. A recent systematic review found that remission of UI after 3 months has a rate up to 86.4 % [13].

11.2 Risk Factors

11.2.1 Maternal Age

Maternal age at first pregnancy seems to correlate with pelvic floor dysfunctions. Leijonhufvud et al. in a cohort study found that incidence rates of POP surgery was 13.8 % among women >30 years old and 6.4 % for younger women [2]. Groutz et al. stated that first vaginal delivery at an older age carries an increased risk for postpartum SUI, with a prevalence of 38.5 % for elderly primiparae (mean age 40) and 9.8 % for young primiparae (mean age 26) [14]. Comparable results come from similar studies [15, 16]. A review published in 2011 concluded that advanced maternal age was an independent risk factor for UI postpartum [17]. In conclusion, young age at first delivery seems to be a protective factor for developing pelvic floor disorders.

11.2.2 Obesity

Gyhagen et al. investigated the prevalence of UI 20 years after childbirth in a big database; in this study maternal body mass index, calculated at early pregnancy, at delivery and 20 years after delivery, was categorized as normal (<25), overweight (>25–29), and obese (<30). In the logistic regression they found an 8 % increased risk of UI per BMI unit increase; the combined effect of vaginal delivery and BMI was substantial, with a risk of 24.7 % with BMI <25 and 54.8 % with BMI >30 [18]. Fornell et al. found that overweight and obesity were strongly associated with urinary incontinence, but not with symptoms of prolapse [19]. Actually there are not randomized clinical trials (RCTs) on weight and UI in association with pregnancy, but from about 20 cohort study we have consistent level 2 of evidence on this association [20].

11.2.3 Biomechanics of Pelvic Floor and Risk Factors Related

Pelvic floor, which is made of both muscles and fasciae, has to sustain the load of abdomen. Hydrostatic load carried by pelvic floor is approximately 40 cm H_2O; if we consider that the average area of female pelvic floor is 94 cm^2, we can estimate the load acting normally to the pelvic floor as 37 N (N) in quiet standing. This one reaches the value of 140 N during a maximum cough and about 90 N during common daily activity. The second stage of labor is particularly important because it lasts about 90 min with uterine contractions: These contractions, lasting about 1 min every 3, develop a load of 54 N, which raises to 120 N during a volitional push. In the cases when obstetric forceps has to be used, the additional force can reach 200 N [21].

It is important to know the mechanisms of damage to the pelvic floor. Up to now, two are the main hypotheses: neurological damage and stretch injury. Levator ani (LA) muscle, which represents the main supporting structure of the pelvic floor, is heavily separated from the mid-line and compressed toward the bone during vaginal delivery, so that a long-lasting stretching damage often follows. Even the attachments of the muscle to the endopelvic fascia and to its connective supports can be impaired and disrupted.

A geometrical model proved that pubococcigeal muscle, the shortest and the most medial muscle of levator ani, is the most damaged one, reaching a stretch ratio of 3.26; muscles injuries occur mainly during the second stage of labor. Kuo-Cheng Lien et al. performed a study developing a computer model to establish the degree of pudendal injury: They found that nerves innervating the anal sphincter are stretched beyond the 15 % strain threshold, and the degree of perineal descent is shown to influence pudendal nerve strain [22]. A biomechanical model was developed to study the structures that, once impaired, can cause urogenital prolapse; in their study Chen et al. showed that the anterior vaginal wall is supported by cardinal and uterosacral ligaments in its upper portion, and by perineal membrane in its lower portion. Under a raised intra-abdominal pressure, the anterior vaginal wall is pushed against the posterior side, supported by the rectum and the levator ani muscle. The biomechanical model showed that the heavier is the pubovisceral impairment, the larger is the anterior wall prolapse, underlying the importance of laevator ani muscle integrity [23].

A prolonged second stage labor is defined as the lack of continuing progress for 3 h with regional anesthesia or 2 h without regional anesthesia, occurring in 11 % of nulliparous women [24, 25]. It can lead to a cesarean delivery or to an operative vaginal delivery (OVD), but randomized clinical trials comparing these techniques are lacking. A cohort study by Crane et al. reported that the mode of delivery does not impact pelvic floor function 1 year after delivery, except for bulge symptoms in OVD group [26]. Prolonged second stage was associated with third-degree or fourth-degree perineal lacerations [27]. Gilboa et al. proposed to evaluate the pubic arch angle by transperineal ultrasound during prolonged second stage to decide delivery mode [28].

Perineal lacerations are strongly associated with pelvic floor damage; in their study Aytan et all showed that episiotomy is an independent predictors for certain POP-Q indices, but had no influence on overall POP-Q stage [29]; the role of medio-lateral episiotomy (MLE) seems to be contradictory: In their retrospective study involving 108 patients Cam et al. found that medio-lateral episiotomy seems to prevent central defects on the anterior vaginal wall, and in this sense it could be preferable to traditional median episiotomy [30]; Sartore et al. found that MLE does not protect against urinary and anal incontinence and genital prolapse and is associated with a lower pelvic floor muscle strength compared with spontaneous perineal lacerations and with more dyspareunia and perineal pain [31].

11.2.4 Fetus Related Factors

Two fetus characteristics have been studied in relation with pelvic organ damage: Fetus weight and fetus head circumference (HC). In their study Lavy et al. calculated cut-off values for risk of levator ani (LA) injury: The relative risk to develop LA trauma is doubled when the head circumference (HC) is ≥35 cm, and it increases to almost 3.5 when the HC is ≥35.5 cm [32]. Eftekhar et al. established that a fetal weight greater than 3,000 g can be considered a factor significantly associated with postpartum SUI [33].

11.2.5 Changes in Extracellular Matrix

The endopelvic fascia is essentially made of collagen and elastin. Pregnancy induces some changes in properties of the vaginal wall; Rahn et al. performed a study on biomechanical properties in mice: They showed augmented distensibility and decreased stiffness [34]. Some important studies performed in mice showed that there are two important proteins involved in prolapse pathogenesis: Fibulin-5 and metalloproteinase 9 (MMP9). Fibulin-5 is essential for the production of normal elastic fibers; it is also important because inhibits the activation of MMP9, involved in prolapse pathogenesis [35]. In presence of stress, fibroblasts, which are mechanosensitive, are able to repair collagen damages, but they need the presence of hormones: Their lack in post menopause could explain prolapse progression [36]. This finding is confirmed by Goepel et al.: In their study, they analyzed the composition of arterial artery comparing 13 women with prolapse with 8 controls; they found that women with prolapse had weaker immunoreactivity to type VI collagen and elastin, and a stronger immunostaining for type III collagen: Particularly, their conclusion was that the changes in the extracellular matrix are only an effect and not the cause of POP [37].

11.3 Consequences

In a recent work, De Lancey highlighted the need for prevention of pelvic floor dysfunctions, considering that reaching a goal of 25 % prevention could save about 30,000 women from this pathology. Particularly he focused on saying that vaginal birth represents the major opportunity for prevention [38]. A spontaneous resolution without surgery is possible: regarding urinary incontinence, Wesnes et al. in a cohort study, found that for each kilogram of weight loss from delivery to 6 months postpartum among women who were incontinent during pregnancy, the relative risk for

UI decreased 2.1 % [39]. Prevention seems to represent the best opportunity: in a recent review wesnes divided into grade of recommandation and level of evidence the things to do for avoiding UI during pregnancy, delivery and post-partum for primary prevention of PFD and as shown in Table 11.1 [20] Lavy et al. proposed a flowchart to address to vaginal delivery or cesarean section according with risk factors, as shown in Table 11.2 [32]. Jelovsek proposed a nomogram to individuate women likely to develop postpartum UI and fecal incontinence, to facilitate decision making in their prevention [40]. Wilson et al. proposed a score system to provide future mothers about the risk of future pelvic floor dysfunction [41]. Concluding, prevention of risk factors seems to represent the best management to pelvic-organ prolapse and UI after childbirth: Many models have been proposed, but without reaching a great popularity and their application seems to lack in many centers in the developed world.

Table 11.1 Recommendation for avoiding UI during pregnancy, delivery and post-partum

	Grade of recommendation	Level of evidence
Actions before pregnancy		
Stop smoking	B	2
Age (<35 at pregnancy)	A	2
Overweight reduction	A	2
Actions during pregnancy		
Reducing constipation	B	2
Stop smoking	D	2, 3
Reducing caffeine	D	–
Crossed legs when coughing	D	–
Bladder training	D	–
Physical activity	B	1, 2
Pelvic floor muscle training	A	1
Restricted weight gain	D	2, 3
Perineal massage	D	–
Actions in association with delivery and postpartum		
Pushing during second stage of labor	D	–
Avoid prolonged second stage of labor	D	2, 3
Restriction of epidural	D	–
Restrictive episiotomy	D	–
Avoid Sphincter tear	D	–
Delivery position	D	–
Restriction of vaginal delivery	D	–
Use of perineal warm packs	B	–
Cesarean section	D	1, 2, 3
Pelvic floor muscle training	A	1
Vaginal cones and electrical stimulation	D	–
Weight reduction (as prepregnancy in 6 months)	B	2
Reducing constipation	C	3

Table 11.2 Flowchart for primary prevention of PFD and to address to vaginal delivery or cesarean section according with risk factors

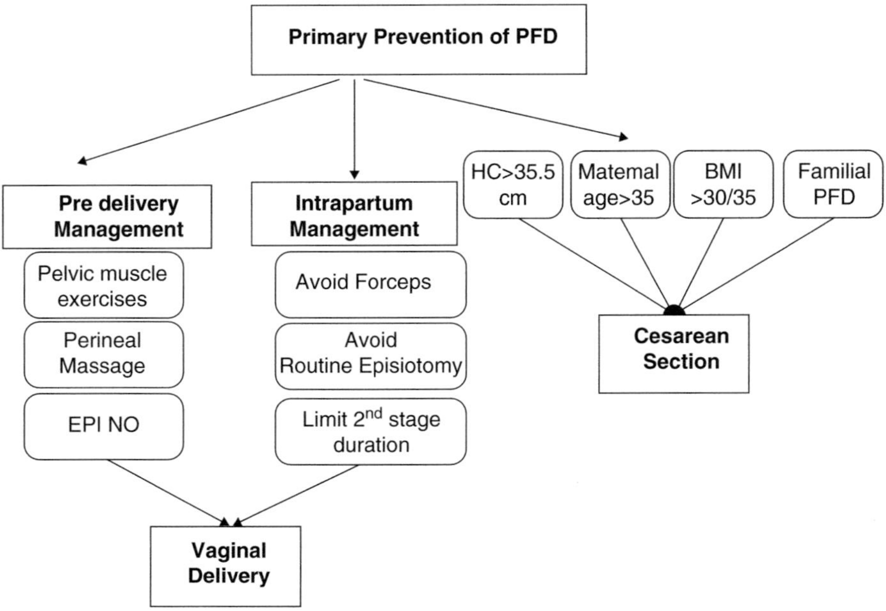

HC-Head Circumference

PFD-Pelvic Fbor Disorder

EPINO-Silicon Inflatable Perineal Dilator

References

1. Glazener C, Elders A, Macarthur C, Lancashire RJ, Herbison P, Hagen S, Dean N, Bain C, Toozs-Hobson P, Richardson K, McDonald A, McPherson G, Wilson D, ProLong Study Group (2013) Childbirth and prolapse: long-term associations with the symptoms and objective measurement of pelvic organ prolapse. BJOG 120(2):161–168
2. Leijonhufvud Å, Lundholm C, Cnattingius S, Granath F, Andolf E, Altman D (2012) Risk of surgically managed pelvic floor dysfunction in relation to age at first delivery. Am J Obstet Gynecol 207(4):303.e1–7
3. Elenskaia K, Thakar R, Sultan AH, Scheer I, Onwude J (2013) Effect of childbirth on pelvic organ support and quality of life: a longitudinal cohort study. Int Urogynecol J 24(6):927–937
4. Chaliha C (2009) Postpartum pelvic floor trauma. Curr Opin Obstet Gynecol 21:474–479
5. Patel DA, Xu X, Thomason AD, Ransom SB, Ivy JS, DeLancey JO (2006) Childbirth and pelvic floor dysfunction: an epidemiologic approach to the assessment of prevention opportunities at delivery. Am J Obstet Gynecol 195(1):23–28, Epub 2006 Mar 30
6. Durnea CM, Khashan AS, Kenny LC, Durnea UA, Smyth MM, O'Reilly BA (2014) Prevalence, etiology and risk factors of pelvic organ prolapse in premenopausal primiparous women. Int Urogynecol J 25:1463–1470

7. Klein MC (2012) Cesarean section on maternal request: a societal and professional failure and symptom of a much larger problem. Birth 39:305
8. Okonkwo NS, Ojengbede OA, Morhason-Bello IO, Adedokun BO (2012) Maternal demand for cesarean section: perception and willingness to request by Nigerian antenatal clients. Int J Womens Health 4:141
9. Burgio KL, Zyczynski H, Locher JL, Richter HE, Redden DT, Wright KC (2003) Urinary incontinence in the 12-month postpartum period. Obstet Gynecol 102:1291
10. Chang SR, Chen KH, Lin HH, Lin MI, Chang TC, Lin WA (2014) Association of mode of delivery with urinary incontinence and changes in urinary incontinence over the first year postpartum. Obstet Gynecol 123(3):568–577
11. Barbosa AM, Marini G, Piculo F, Rudge CV, Calderon IM, Rudge MV (2013) Prevalence of urinary incontinence and pelvic floor muscle dysfunction in primiparae two years after cesarean section: cross-sectional study. Sao Paulo Med J 131(2):95–99
12. Chan SS, Cheung RY, Yiu KW, Lee LL, Chung TK (2013) Prevalence of urinary and fecal incontinence in Chinese women during and after their first pregnancy. Int Urogynecol J 24(9):1473–1479
13. Cerruto MA, D'Elia C, Aloisi A, Fabrello M, Artibani W (2013) Prevalence, incidence and obstetric factors' impact on female urinary incontinence in Europe: a systematic review. Urol Int 90(1):1–9
14. Groutz A, Helpman L, Gold R, Pauzner D, Lessing JB, Gordon D (2007) First vaginal delivery at an older age: does it carry an extra risk for the development of stress urinary incontinence? Neurourol Urodyn 26(6):779–782
15. Kuh D, Cardozo L, Hardy R (1999) Urinary incontinence in middle-aged women: childhood enuresis and other lifetime risk factors in a British prospective cohort. J. Epidemiol, Community Health
16. Foldspang A, Mommsen S, Lam GW, Elving L (1992) Parity as a correlate of adult female urinary incontinence prevalence. Epidemiol Community Health 46(6):595–600
17. Hijaz A, Sadeghi Z, Byrne L et al (2012) Advanced maternal age as a risk factor for stress urinary incontinence: a review of the literature. Int Urogynecol J 23:395–401
18. Gyhagen M, Bullarbo M, Nielsen TF, Milsom I (2013) The prevalence of urinary incontinence 20 years after childbirth: a national cohort study in singleton primiparae after vaginal or caesarean delivery. BJOG 120(2):144–151
19. Uustal Fornell E, Wingren G, Kjølhede P (2004) Factors associated with pelvic floor dysfunction with emphasis on urinary and fecal incontinence and genital prolapse: an epidemiological study. Acta Obstet Gynecol Scand 83(4):383–389
20. Wesnes SL, Lose G (2013) Preventing urinary incontinence during pregnancy and postpartum: a review. Int Urogynecol J 24(6):889–899
21. Ashton-Miller JA, Delancey JO (2009) On the biomechanics of vaginal birth and common sequelae. Annu Rev Biomed Eng 11:163–176
22. Lien KC, Morgan DM, Delancey JO, Ashton-Miller JA (2005) Pudendal nerve stretch during vaginal birth: a 3D computer simulation. Am J Obstet Gynecol 192(5):1669–1676
23. Chen L, Ashton-Miller JA, Hsu Y, DeLancey JO (2006) Interaction among apical support, levator ani impairment, and anterior vaginal wall prolapse. Obstet Gynecol 108(2):324–332
24. American College of Obstetrics and Gynecology Committee on Practice Bulletins-Obstetrics (2003) ACOG Practice Bulletin, Number 49, December 2003 Dystocia and augmentation of labor. Obstet Gynecol 102(6):1445–1454
25. Menticoglou SM, Mannin F, Harman C, Morrison I (1995) Perinatal outcome in relation to second-stage duration. Am J Obstet Gynecol 173:906–912
26. Crane AK, Geller EJ, Bane H, Ju R, Myers E, Matthews CA (2013) Evaluation of pelvic floor symptoms and sexual function in primiparous women who underwent operative vaginal delivery versus cesarean delivery for second-stage arrest. Female Pelvic Med Reconstr Surg 19(1):13–16
27. Laughon SK, Berghella V, Reddy UM, Sundaram R, Lu Z, Hoffman MK (2014) Neonatal and maternal outcomes with prolonged second stage of labor. Obstet Gynecol 124(1):57–67

28. Gilboa Y, Kivilevitch Z, Spira M, Kedem A, Katorza E, Moran O, Achiron R (2013) Pubic arch angle in prolonged second stage of labor: clinical significance. Ultrasound Obstet Gynecol 41(4):442–446
29. Aytan H, Tok EC, Ertunc D, Yasa O (2014) The effect of episiotomy on pelvic organ prolapse assessed by pelvic organ prolapse quantification system. Eur J Obstet Gynecol Reprod Biol 173:34–37
30. Cam C, Asoglu MR, Selcuk S, Aran T, Tug N, Karateke A (2012) Does mediolateral episiotomy decrease central defects of the anterior vaginal wall? Arch Gynecol Obstet 285(2):411–415
31. Sartore A, De Seta F, Maso G, Pregazzi R, Grimaldi E, Guaschino S (2004) The effects of mediolateral episiotomy on pelvic floor function after vaginal delivery. Obstet Gynecol 103(4):669–673
32. Lavy Y, Sand PK, Kaniel CI, Hochner-Celnikier D (2012) Can pelvic floor injury secondary to delivery be prevented? Int Urogynecol J 23(2):165–173
33. Eftekhar T, Hajibaratali B, Ramezanzadeh F, Shariat M (2006) Postpartum evaluation of stress urinary incontinence among primiparas. Int J Gynaecol Obstet 94(2):114–118, Epub 2006 Jul 17
34. Rahn DD, Ruff MD, Brown SA, Tibbals HF, Word RA (2008) Biomechanical properties of the vaginal wall: effect of pregnancy, elastic fiber deficiency, and pelvic organprolapse. Am J Obstet Gynecol 198(5):590.e1–6
35. Connell KA (2011) Elastogenesis in the vaginal wall and pelvic-organ prolapse. N Engl J Med 364(24):2356–2358, Connell KA
36. Zong W, Jallah ZC, Stein SE, Abramowitch SD, Moalli PA (2010) Repetitive mechanical stretch increases extracellular collagenase activity in vaginal fibroblasts. Female Pelvic Med Reconstr Surg 16(5):257–262
37. Goepel C, Johanna Kantelhardt E, Karbe I, Stoerer S, Dittmer J (2011) Changes of glycoprotein and collagen immunolocalization in the uterine artery wall of postmenopausal women with and without pelvic organ prolapse. Acta Histochem 113(3):375–381
38. DeLancey JO (2005) The hidden epidemic of pelvic floor dysfunction: achievable goals for improved prevention and treatment. Am J Obstet Gynecol 192(5):1488–1495
39. Wesnes SL, Hunskaar S, Bo K, Rortveit G (2010) Urinary incontinence and weight change during pregnancy and postpartum: a cohort study. Am J Epidemiol 172(9):1034–1044
40. Jelovsek JE, Piccorelli A, Barber MD, Tunitsky-Bitton E, Kattan MW (2013) Prediction models for postpartum urinary and fecal incontinence in primiparous women. Female Pelvic Med Reconstr Surg 19(2):110–118
41. Wilson D, Dornan J, Milsom I, Freeman R (2014) UR-CHOICE: can we provide mothers-to-be with information about the risk of future pelvic floor dysfunction? Int Urogynecol J 25:1449–1452

Fecal Incontinence After Childbirth: Diagnostic and Clinical Aspects

12

Alvise Frasson and Giuseppe Dodi

A huge number of scientific papers highlight that many neuromuscular and soft tissue injuries to the pelvic floor arise after vaginal childbirth, resulting in the development of anal and urinary incontinence and pelvic organ prolapse. Focusing on the posterior compartment, the International Continence Society stated that "anal incontinence (AI) is the involuntary loss of flatus, liquid or solid stool that is a social or hygienic problem."

The reluctance of patients to admit the symptoms of AI, even when following childbirth, makes difficult to establish its true prevalence, which in the literature is reported of about 10–17 % [1–3] in general population, 5–26 % within the first year after vaginal delivery and 17–62 % when women complain a major perineal trauma or have been delivered with forceps [4]. It is likely that this wide range can be linked to a misclassification of the most important etiological factor of AI, when a damage to puboanalis and/or transverse perineii muscles is reported as a sphincter tear, or when there is a wrong identification of the lesion: what could happen is presence of a huge edema or of an abundant blood loss after delivery. This inability to achieve a proper diagnose occurs in 87 % of midwives, 28 % of young doctors, 14 % of physicians, compared to 1 % of experienced clinicians [5]. The above concept means that the lesion indicated as an occult defect of the sphincters, was just an undiagnosed or misclassified tear that could have been correctly diagnosed with a proper training [2]. Furthermore, it is likely that the real percentage of occult tears is less than 1 %: on the contrary transanal ecography demonstrated that a damage of the sphincters can be found in 35 % of symptomatic primiparous women and 13 % of multiparous [6].

A. Frasson • G. Dodi (✉)
Department of Surgery, Oncology and Gastroenterology,
Via Nicolò Giustiniani, 2, Padova, Italy
e-mail: alvise.frasson@unipd.it; giuseppe.dodi@unipd.it

D. Riva, G. Minini (eds.), *Childbirth-Related Pelvic Floor Dysfunction: Risk Factors, Prevention, Evaluation, and Treatment*,
DOI 10.1007/978-3-319-18197-4_12

Potential risk factors for sphincter's injury due to childbirth are first vaginal delivery and multiparity, the use of forceps, episiotomy, a prolonged second stage of labor prolonged by anesthesia, birth weight, shoulder dystocia, and a persistent occipito-posterior position, age, and obesity. Episiotomy may represent a specific iatrogenic damage to the sphincters, mostly when performed in the midline. The wide use of this procedure is not always considered beneficial (see Chap. 10): thus international guidelines indicate to perform it in less than 30 % of patient and to carry out a mediolateral episiotomy to reduce the risk of anal sphincter rupture (12 % vs 2 %) [2, 4].

Focusing on the macroscopic appearance of the damage to the sphincters, Sultan [7, 8] suggested that obstetric injuries resulting from the direct trauma lead to different degrees of damage as reported in Table 12.1 and in the Fig. 12.1. A third- or

Table 12.1 Classification of a macroscopic anal sphincters' damage [7, 8]

First degree	laceration of the vaginal epithelium or perineal skin only
Second degree	involvement of the perineal muscles but not the anal sphincters
Third degree	disruption of the anal sphincter muscles. This should be further subdivided into:
	3a: <50 % thickness of external anal sphincter torn
	3b: >50 % thickness of external anal sphincter torn
	3c: both external and internal anal sphincter
Fourth degree	Third degrees tear with disruption of the rectal mucosa or anal epithelium
An isolated rectal tear without involvement of the anal sphincter is rare and should not be included in the above classification.	

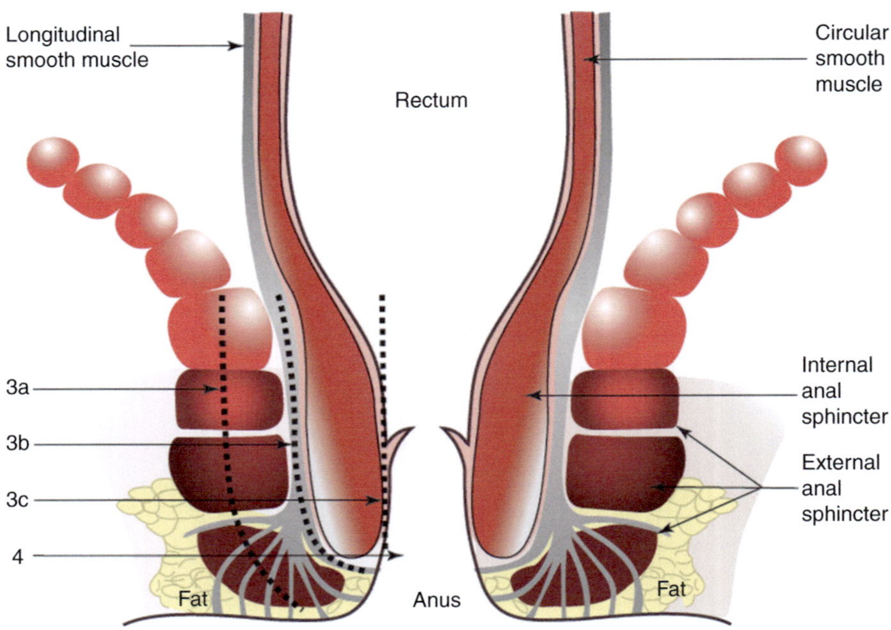

Fig. 12.1 Representation of the anal sphincters and classification of third or fourth perineal tears (Reproduced from Sultan [8])

fourth-*degree sphincter's damage* after childbirth is an almost certain sign and it is highly predictive of a future development of AI, but it is not often recognized at the time of delivery. Even if the direct trauma to the perineal tissue mostly causes a lesion of the sphincters, it may damage the nerves too, when the pudendal nerve at the Alcock's canal or the pelvic branches of the sacral plexus are compressed by the fetal head during childbirth. The signs of the damage will be a delay in the conduction of the nerve, as shown by pudendal nerve terminal motor latency (PNTML) and histological evidence of denervation of the striated pelvic floor muscles. Even the stretching of nervous fibers can temporarily cause symptoms of pudendal neuropathy: recovery from symptoms and normalization of the PNTML in about 60 % of patients within 2 months are common. Histologically, if the lesion is reversible, an increase in sphincter fibers density can be evidenced at about 2 months after delivery, as an expression of reinnervation following denervation. Potential risk factors for pudendal nerve damage are multiparity, forceps delivery, increased duration of the second stage of labor, third- or fourth-degree perineal tears and high birth weight. Apart from AI, if the neuropathy persists, it can cause weakness of the pelvic floor and its related symptomatology [2, 5].

To note, even if the direct trauma to anal sphincter or nerves are known as the most important factor of AI, nevertheless the use of a cesarean delivery does not prevent from AI and its symptoms [2, 9, 10].

12.1 Diagnostic Steps

It is mandatory that physicians perform a full assessment of patients including medical history, general physical examination and proctological examination, instrumental studies, with the aim of fully outline AI's characteristics.

12.1.1 Medical History

The history must not be focused only on AI, but rather to retrieve all patient's medical informations concerning systemic disorders and co-morbidities as urinary incontinence, previous surgery (mainly on the posterior compartment and gynecological procedures), spinal injuries, parity, drugs, and lifestyle. Moreover, the patient should be questioned on bowel function and on bowel care including diet, fluid intake and laxatives, and how these influence AI. Then, the symptoms experienced by the patient must be investigated and pointed out just like every kind of AI or other conditions which cause soiling (e.g., fistulas, external hemorrhoids, anal, or low rectal tumors). If the patient describes an AI only for liquid stool, then a colonic cause of diarrhea should be excluded. If an AI is present, it must be differentiated as a flatus incontinence, passive leakage, or urge incontinence (Table 12.2), never forgetting that an overlapping between these conditions is always possible. Furthermore, the need of pads, duration, frequency and timing of AI's episodes must be outlined. Hence, the severity of AI can be graduated as: (a) minor, if incontinence happens less than once a month; (b) moderate, if incontinence to solids happens more than once a month or to liquids more than once a week; (c) severe, when incontinence to

Table 12.2 Types of anal incontinence

Type	Description	Defect
Flatus incontinence	Incontinence of flatus due to inability to differentiate gas from solid or liquid	Internal anal sphincter
Passive leakage	Involuntary soiling or discharge of liquid or solid stool without patient awareness	Internal anal sphincter
Urge incontinence	Inability to retain feces as long as needed to find a toilet once the need to defecate is perceived	External anal sphincter

Table 12.3 The Wexner score [11]

	Frequency				
Type of incontinence	Never	Rarely	Sometimes	Usually	Always
Solid	0	1	2	3	4
Liquid	0	1	2	3	4
Gas	0	1	2	3	4
Wears pad	0	1	2	3	4
Lifestyle alteration	0	1	2	3	4

Never, 0; rarely, <1/month; sometimes, <1/week; ≥ 1/month; usually. <1/day, ≥1/week; always, ≥1/day
0, perfect; 20, complete incontinence

Table 12.4 The American Medical Systems (AMS) score [12]

Over the past 4 weeks, how often:	Never	Rarely	Sometimes	Weekly	Daily	Several times daily
Did you experience accidental bowel leakage of gas?	0	1	7	13	19	25
Did you experience minor bowel soiling or seepage?	0	31	37	43	49	55
Did you experience significant accidental bowel leakage of liquid stool?	0	61	73	85	97	109
Did you experience significant accidental bowel leakage of solid stool?	0	67	79	91	103	115
Has this accidental leakage affected your lifestyle?	0	1	2	3	4	5

Several times daily, >1 episode a day; daily, 1 episode a day; weekly, 1 or more episodes a week but <1 a day; sometimes, >1 episode in the past 4 weeks but <1 a week; rarely, 1 episode in the past 4 weeks; never, 0 episodes in the past 4 weeks

solids and/or liquids happens daily or several times a week. All these characteristics can be better classified with grading systems as the *Wexner score system* (Table 12.3) or the *American Medical Systems (AMS) score* (Table 12.4), which allows to use an objective parameter to evaluate AI, to verify the response to therapy and to follow up its evolution.

Last but not least, it is of enormous relevance to question the patients, possibly with questionnaires such as the SF-36, on restrictions, quality of life, satisfaction, needs, sexual dysfunction, and on how AI influences them [1–3].

12.1.2 Clinical Examination

The proctological examination should start from the inspection of the perineum and anus checking their integrity and looking for scar from previous surgery or episiotomies, absence of the perineal body, a keyhole deformity of the anus suggesting a sphincter defect, or just for irritation or excoriation of the skin due to soiling. Moreover, during the inspection one should ask the patient to strain in order to check the presence of a descending perineum or of mucosal, hemorrhoidal or full-thickness rectal prolapse. Then, the digital rectal examination verifies the sphincter tone at rest (indicative of internal anal sphincter function), in contraction (indicative of external anal sphincter function) and during squeezing, the latter to check the function of the puborectalis muscle which with squeezing should push the examiner's finger anteriorly. Asking the patient to cough will result in an external sphincter contraction, thus checking the anal sphincter reflex. The rectal examination may show an asymmetry of the sphincter suggesting a regional defect. Finally, a proctoscopy and a rectosigmoidoscopy with a rigid instrument must be done to complete the proctological visit.

12.1.3 Instrumental Devices

(a) *Transanal ultrasonography*: nowadays, depending on the grade of the sphincter lesions, the surgeon will chose different techniques to repair it. Hence, the use of transanal ultrasonography is necessary to study the muscle and its damage in order to plan the therapeutic program. This type of examination studies all the layers of the anorectal canal, obviously including the possible defects of the puborectalis muscle, levator ani muscle, internal and external sphincter. Concerning the sphincter defects Starck proposed the use of a useful score system to classify the injuries, with values ranging from 0 (no muscular defect) to 16 (defect >180° involving the whole length and depth of the muscle) (Table 12.5). The prevalence of symptoms of incontinence in primiparous women is reported being 5–26 % within the 1st year following vaginal delivery: with the use of endoanal ultrasound the percentage of damage of the sphincters is shown in up to 35 % of uniparous and 13 % of multiparous [1, 2, 6].

(b) *Electromyography (EMG)*: both single fiber and concentric needle EMG studies the integrity of the external anal sphincter and how the contraction changes the electrical activity of the sphincter and of levator ani muscle. This technique has been used in the diagnostical setting for investigate AI's etiology until the advent of ultrasound, which is a simpler procedure. Now the major indication for EMG is anismus and scientific speculations. (For anal sphincter surface EMG see Chap. 6).

Table 12.5 Starck's scoring system for the endoultrasonography classification of sphincters' injuries [23]

Defect characteristic	Score 0	Score 1	Score 2	Score 3
Internal sphincter defect				
Length	None	Half or less	More than half	Whole
Depth	None	Partial	Total	–
Size	None	≤90°	91–180°	>180°
External sphincter defect				
Length	None	Half or less	More than half	Whole
Depth	None	Partial	Total	–
Size	None	≤90°	91–180°	> 180°

(c) *Pudendal nerve terminal motor latency (PNTML)*: this technique studies the time to contraction due to a stimulation to the pudendal nerve. Although PNTML is often prolonged in patients with AI, its clinical value has been questioned because of the low predictive value, the poor sensitivity and specificity in discriminating muscle and nerve injury, the poor correlation with symptoms. Thus up to now is less and less carried out [1, 2].

(d) *Anorectal manometry*: this exam allows a full investigation of sphincters' function and rectal characteristics: (1) anal sphincter pressure, (2) rectal sensation: perception of fecal mass distending the rectal wall at the lowest volume that evocates the first sensation of a mass (a), or at the volume at which there is the need to defecate (b), or at the maximum volume tolerated (c), (3) rectoanal reflexes: the rectoanal inhibitory reflex – RAIR – is the inhibition of the internal anal sphincter tone with a distension of the rectum, (4) rectal compliance: adaptation of rectum to the incoming stool checking the different values at rest (showing the tonic function of both the internal and external anal sphincter), during voluntary contraction and during Valsalva or cough (external anal sphincter function). Patients with AI have a low resting pressure (defect of the internal anal sphincter), a low squeeze pressure and a low duration of squeezing time (external anal sphincter dysfunction → inability to suppress defecation). Moreover, an alteration of the rectal sensation may contribute to AI by a misunderstanding of the presence of stool and of the need to defecate. Urge AI could be linked to a decrease in rectal compliance which may cause an increased frequency of defecation and a rapid transit of stool through the rectum. While manometry looks as a promising technique, its clinical utility is limited by the low standardization of the procedure and the low sensitivity and specificity in the discrimination of continent and incontinent patients [1, 2].

(e) *Balloon rectal test*: a quick and simple test useful in outpatients is the balloon rectal test which allows to evidence the rectal sensitivity and compliance. A balloon has to be placed in the rectum (Fig. 12.2) to mimic the presence of stool: its gradual inflation with air or fluid will allow to measure the volume of the following items (Table 12.6): (1) first sensation; (2) desire to defecate; (3) urgency to defecation; (4) pain. In incontinent patients values are lower than normal (rectal hypersensitivity). Higher values indicate a rectal hyposensitivity.

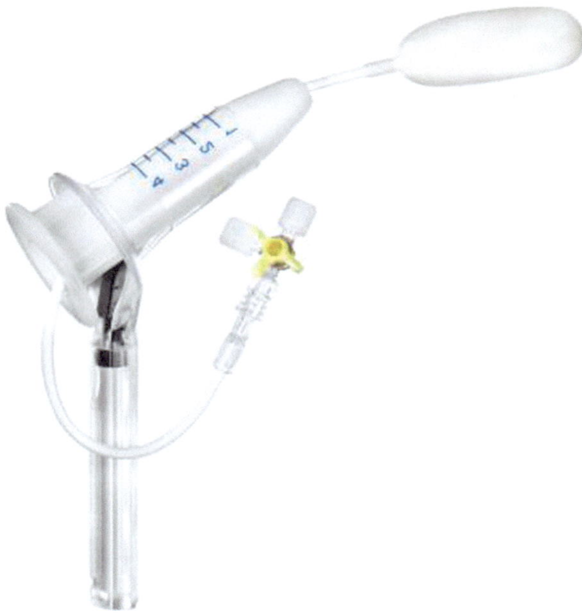

Fig. 12.2 Multi-Functional Anoscope (MFA – Sapi Med SPA): an anoscope addicted with a balloon that can be used to measure rectal sensitivity and compliance

Table 12.6 Values of the parameters checked with the inflation of an endorectal balloon

Parameters	Normal value
First sensation	30–60 cc of air or fluid
Defecatory desire volume	60–160 cc of air or fluid
Maximum tolerable volume	160–270 cc of air or fluid
Pain	>270

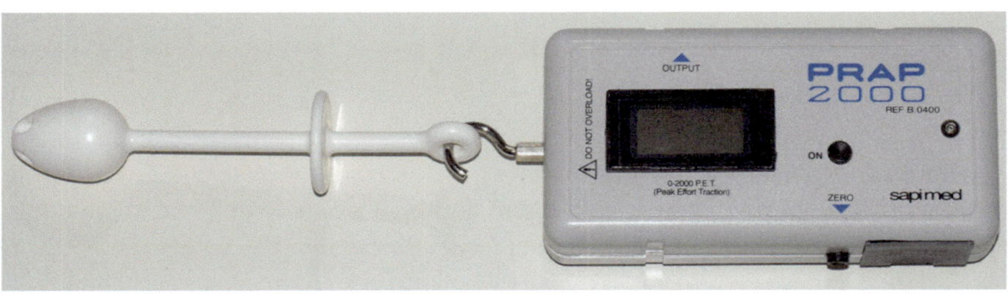

Fig. 12.3 Digital dynamometer PRAP2000 with solid disposable sphere (Sapi Med S.P.A.)

(f) *Solid sphere test* [13–15]: this is a quick and painless procedure to check rectal sensitivity on outpatients as a step preliminary to further investigation. A solid sphere is introduced into the anal canal and is attached to a digital dynamometer (Fig. 12.3) to quantify the resistance of the sphincters to the extraction of the sphere. First, the patient must contract the sphincter (voluntary contraction phase), then strain to eject it (ejection phase), finally at rest the sphere must be pulled out (baseline phase) (Table 12.7). This test allows to differentiate the

Table 12.7 Normal value checked with the solid sphere test

Parameters	Normal value
Voluntary contraction	1,000–1,200 g
Baseline	200–400 g
Ejection	Ideally 0 g or anyway less than at baseline

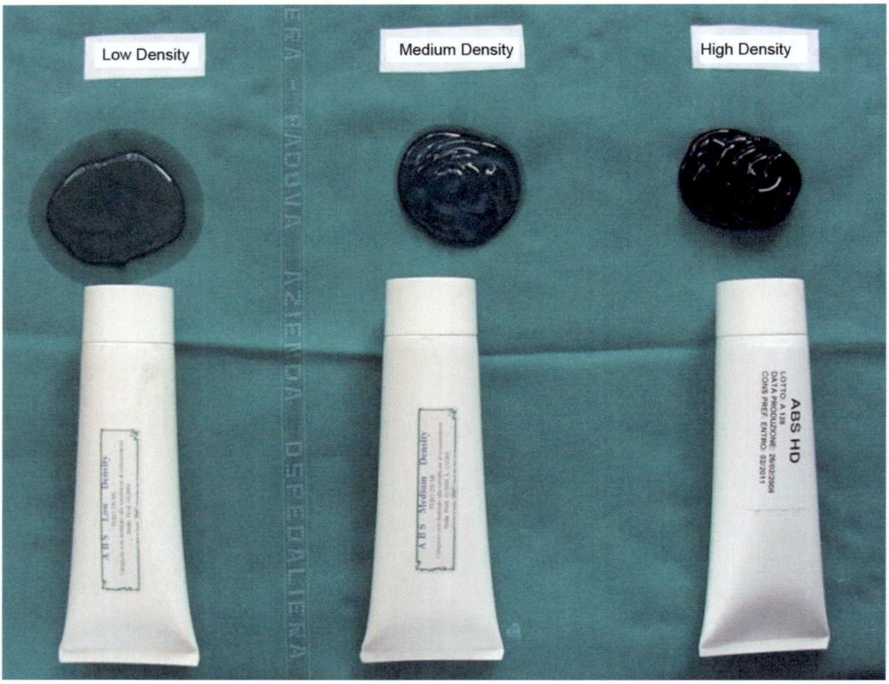

Fig. 12.4 Artificial blue stool (ABS): from left to right the low, the medium and the high-density blue gel (Sapi Med S.P.A.)

internal sphincter's activity at rest from the external sphincter's activity during contraction. Moreover, it is possible to highlight a paradoxical contraction or a failure of relaxation of the puborectalis muscle when the patient is asked to strain. All these parameters are easily checked on an outpatient basis being easily correlated with anorectal manometry, EMG and defecography data.

(g) *Artificial blue stool*: the aim of this test is to check the patient's ability to retain feces. This procedure can be done in outpatients by filling the rectum with a blue gel which mimics stool (Fig. 12.4). This gel is available in three different densities: high, medium, and low density. The exam is started with the high-density gel. After filling the rectum with it the patient is asked to do some physical activity and then checked for any incontinence: if negative, the patient undergoes a stress test with a small enema. If negative again, the patient will be checked with the medium density gel as described before and, if needed, with the low density one. The test is useful to compare the results after therapy.

12.2 Treatment

There are many options to cure fecal incontinence, the surgical treatment being reported to achieve better long-lasting results. Options other than surgery are the conservative medical therapy, behavioral therapy or training of the pelvic floor muscles, neurosacral modulation.

12.2.1 Medical Therapy, Pelvic Floor Muscle Therapy (PFMT), and Behavioral Therapy

A conservative treatment with drugs which increase stool consistency and prolong colonic transit time should be the first line therapy as it could be effective in a discrete number of patients [5]. Moreover other types of first line treatments, associated or not to medical therapy, are the *PFMT* and behavioral therapy. Both achieve lower incontinence rates during pregnancy and at 1 year of follow-up while this result does not persist in the long-term, likely because of subsequent pregnancies or of the discontinuation of PFMT or biofeedback. Stimulating women to undergo PFMT and biofeedback during pregnancy and even after, it is essential to achieve long-term good results [4, 5, 16].

12.2.2 Surgical Treatment

Sphincter's repair is the main surgical treatment of AI as its damage represents the main cause of incontinence. An immediate repair of the sphincter's defect performed within 24 h from childbirth is to be preferred because it has been demonstrated that it is associated with less risk of fecal urgency and better long-term results if compared to delayed sphincteroplasty [2, 17, 18]. The primary repair reduces bleeding, edema, and the likelihood of infection, which is in itself a cause of early failure. Gynecologists prefer the *end-to-end technique*, general surgeon the overlapping procedure that can be performed only if the external sphincter has a full-thickness damage. Following Sultan's paper in 1999 [19] that showed a better outcome with the *overlapping technique* [2, 5, 18, 20], other authors have compared the immediate end-to-end technique to the overlapping repair: the latter appears to deserve better results within 12 months, while at 36 months the difference between the techniques seems to decrease [16, 17].

An exhaustive examination of the pelvic floor to clearly classify injuries and to repair damages to the vaginal mucosa and rectovaginal septum is mandatory before approaching the posterior compartment with a reconstructive surgery. Through a curved perineal incision anterior to the anus, the internal and external anal sphincters' defects are addressed with the aim of recognizing and repairing separately the injury of the internal anal sphincter with interrupted 3–0 or 4–0 sutures in delayed absorbable monofilament. The separated repair of the internal sphincter is preferable as it has been reported to reduce the risk of AI [5, 17–21]; otherwise the internal anal sphincter will be repaired in a single layer with the external one. The external

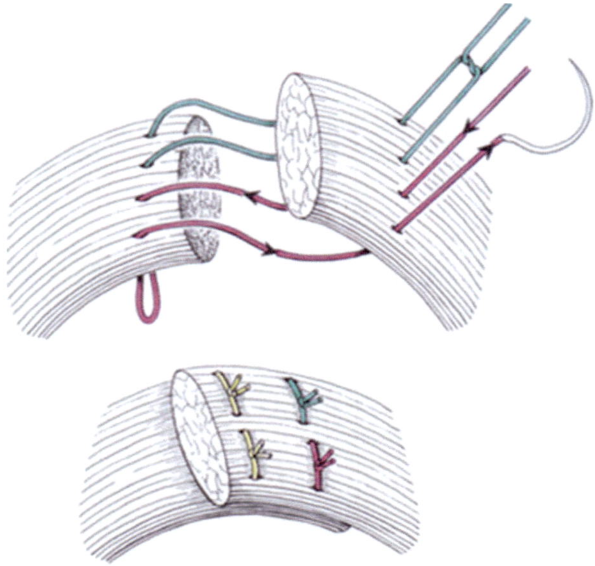

Fig. 12.5 Representation of the overlap technique (From Aigmuller et al. [21])

sphincter can be recognized as a striated muscle with retracted and fibrotic edges; they must be pulled one toward the other with two Allis clamp. If an end-to-end technique is performed the edges of the sphincter are approximated with interrupted sutures in delayed absorbable 2-0 monofilament to allow an adequate consolidation of the scar. Otherwise, the overlapping technique requires a wide dissection, at least 2 cm deep, of the two edges of the sphincter with scissors, in order to achieve an adequate surfacing area for the overlapping. Three interrupted stitches are needed to approximate the muscle's edges, passing from the top of the superior flap through the sphincter down to its bottom and back, making the proximal end of the superior flap lying on the distal portion of the inferior one and vice versa (Fig. 12.5), always with an absorbable delayed monofilament suture. Anyhow, in performing the end-to-end technique or the overlapping one, the fibrotic edges of the sphincter should be included within the sutures.

The trauma induced by childbirth may also cause damage to perineal skin, vaginal mucosa, perineal muscle, and anorectal mucosa too. Hence, apart from the initial repair of the mucosa and the subsequent sphincter's reconstruction, an associated anterior levator ani plication may be required: it is performed through an incision posterior to the anus (postanal repair), suturing puborectalis and pubococcygeus muscles. The tears of the perineum are repaired layer by layer. At the end of the reconstructive phase an examination of the anorectum to exclude unrecognized injuries or an iatrogenic perforation of the anorectal mucosa is mandatory.

Whenever the sphincter's defect is unrecognized at time of delivery or the primary repair has failed, a secondary sphincter repair can be performed at least 3 months later. This procedure is usually performed by a colorectal surgeon with an overlapping technique. Generally at time of a secondary repair the internal sphincter is not easily recognized and thus repaired in a single layer with the external sphincter. An isolated internal sphincter defect is not usually repaired. [5, 20]

Whether it is a primary or a secondary repair and even if the overlap technique has better results, guidelines and papers suggest that an end-to-end or an overlap procedure can be performed at discretion of each surgeon but with the recommendation that if possible the internal sphincter is repaired separately and that the surgeon or gynecologist is appropriately trained in these procedures [2, 17, 18, 20, 21].

An early relapse of AI can be due to hematomas, wound infections, inappropriate experience of the physician, lack of a tension free repair or another unrecognized sphincter defect.

Whenever the sphincteroplasty does not improve AI or if the damage to the sphincter, perineum and nerves is too extensive, another feasible procedure is the creation of a neosphincter with a *dynamic graciloplasty*. This technique requires the detachment of the distal two third of the gracilis muscle from the thigh and its transposition and rotation to surround the anus. Care must be taken to preserve its neurovascular bundle where an electrical stimulator is placed to maintain a continuous contraction and thus continence. Hence, the defecation is obtained by turning off the stimulation. Improvement of continence has been reported in 60 to 85% of patients and persists up to 24 months in 66 % [5, 22].

Another option to improve AI is the *neurosacral modulation*. This procedure is a standardized technique to cure idiopathic AI and it has been demonstrated to improve incontinence even in women affected by complete rupture of the internal and external anal sphincter after childbirth. The improvement of AI seems to be quite similar to patient with an intact sphincter and to persist longer than any surgical repair of the sphincter. Thus, considering that this technique does not avoid a subsequent surgical reconstruction of the sphincters, that there is no possibility to damage the sphincters and the low morbidity of the procedure, is nowadays an option to be considered in the cure of postpartum incontinence [5, 22].

In case of failure of all the above techniques and the patient complains of a bad quality of life, a fecal diversion may be performed [5, 22].

References

1. Ratto C, Doglietto GB (eds) (2007) Fecal incontinence diagnosis and treatmen. Springer, Berlin/Heidelberg/New York
2. Abrams P, Cardozo L, Khoury S, Wein A (eds) (2009) Incontinence. 4th international consultation on incontinence, paris, 5–8 july 2008. Health Publications Ltd, Portsmouth
3. Abrams P, Andersson KE, Birder L, Brubaker L, Cardozo L, Chapple C, Cottenden A, Davila W, de Ridder D, Dmochowski R, Drake M, Dubeau C, Fry C, Hanno P, Smith JH, Herschorn S, Hosker G, Kelleher C, Koelbl H, Khoury S, Madoff R, Milsom I, Moore K, Newman D, Nitti V, Norton C, Nygaard I, Payne C, Smith A, Staskin D, Tekgul S, Thuroff J, Tubaro A, Vodusek D, Wein A, Wyndaele JJ, Members of Committees, Fourth International Consultation on Incontinence (2010) Fourth International Consultation on Incontinence Recommendations of the International Scientific Committee: Evaluation and treatment of urinary incontinence, pelvic organ prolapse, and fecal incontinence. Neurourol Urodyn 29:213–240. doi:10.1002/nau.20870

4. Boyle R, Hay-Smith EJC, Cody JD, Mørkved S (2012) Pelvic floor muscle training for prevention and treatment of urinary and faecal incontinence in antenatal and postnatal women. Cochrane Database Syst Rev (10):CD007471. doi:10.1002/14651858.CD007471.pub2
5. Dudding TC, Vaizey CJ, Kamm MA (2008) Obstetric anal sphincter injury: incidence, risk factors, and management. Ann Surg 247:224–237. doi:10.1097/SLA.0b013e318142cdf4
6. Santoro G, Wieczorek AP, Bartram CI (eds) (2010) Pelvic floor disorders, imaging and multidisciplinary approach to management. Springer, Berlin/Heidelberg/New York
7. Sultan AH (1999) Clinical focus: obstetric perineal injury and faecal incontinence after childbirth – editorial: obstetrical perineal injury and anal incontinence. Clinical Risk 5:193–196
8. Sultan AH, Thakar R (2007) Third and fourth degree tears. In: Sultan AH, Thakar R, Fenner D (eds) Perineal and anal sphincter trauma. Springer, London, pp 33–51
9. Nelson RL, Furner SE, Westercamp M, Farquhar C (2010) Cesarean delivery for the prevention of anal incontinence. Cochrane Database Syst Rev (2): CD006756. doi:10.1002/14651858.CD006756.pub2
10. Pretlove S, Thompson P, Toozs-Hobson P, Radley S, Khan K (2008) Does the mode of delivery predispose women to anal incontinence in the first year postpartum? a comparative systematic review. BJOG 115:421–434
11. Jorge JMN, Wexner SD (1993) Etiology and management of fecal incontinence. Dis Colon Rectum 36:77–97
12. Vaizey CJ, Carapeti E, Cahill JA, Kamm MA (1999) Prospective comparison of faecal incontinence grading systems. Gut 44:77–80
13. Cavallari F, Dodi G (2004) Test della sfera solida: validazione metodologica e dati preliminari nella stipsi da anismo. Pelvi Perineologia 23:132–135
14. Guerette N, Neimark M, Kopka SL, Jones JE, Davila GW (2004) Initial experience with a new method for the dynamic assessment of pelvic floor function in women: the Kolpexin Pull Test. Int Urogynecol J Pelvic Floor Dysfunct 15:39–43
15. Azpiroz F, Enck P, Whitehead WE (2002) Anorectal functional testing: review of collective experience. Am J Gastroenterol 97:232–240
16. Glazener CMA, MacArthur C, Hagen S, Elders A, Lancashire R, Herbison GP, Wilson PD (2014) Twelve-year follow-up of conservative management of postnatal urinary and faecal incontinence and prolapse outcomes: randomised controlled trial. BJOG 121:112–120
17. Fernando RJ, Sultan AH, Kettle C, Thakar R (2013) Methods of repair for obstetric anal sphincter injury. Cochrane Database Syst Rev (12):CD002866. doi:10.1002/14651858.CD002866.pub3
18. Fernando RJ (2005) Anal sphincter injury at childbirth – *i*mmediate or delayed repair? overlapping or end-to-end technique? midline or mediolateral episiotomy? plus: risk factors, and tactics for subsequent deliveries. OBG Management 17:22–39
19. Sultan AH, Monga AK, Kumar D, Stanton SL (1999) Primary repair of obstetric anal sphincter rupture using the overlap technique. Br J Obstet Gynaecol 106:318–323
20. Royal College of Obstetricians and Gynecologists, Fernando RJ, Williams AA, Adams EJ (2007) The management of third- and fourth-degree perineal tears (Green-top Guideline No. 29). http://www.rcog.org.uk/files/rcog-corp/GTG2911022011.pdf
21. Aigmueller T, Umek W, Elenskaia K, Frudinger A, Pfeifer J, Helmer H, Huemer H, Tammaa A, Van der Kleyn M, Tamussino K, Koelle D, Austrian Urogynecology Working Group (2013) Guidelines for the management of third and fourth degree perineal tears after vaginal birth from the Austrian Urogynecology Working Group. Int Urogynecol J 24:553–558
22. Whitehead WE, Wald A, Norton NJ (2001) Treatment options for fecal incontinence. Dis Colon Rectum 44:131–144
23. Starck M, Bohe M, Valentin L (2003) Results of endosonographic imaging of the anal sphincter 2–7 days after primary repair of third or fourth-degree obstetric sphincter tears. Ultrasound Obstet Gynecol 22:609–615

Principles and Methods of Physiotherapy After Delivery

13

Simonetta Minoli

13.1 Introduction

According to a number of epidemiological studies, one of the most socially devastating sequels of vaginal delivery is pelvic floor muscle's damage [1]. It can cause pelvic organ prolapse with loss of bladder and bowel control, making life very hard to manage and painful: child-care, walking, sitting, sleeping, and human relationships may become problematic [2, 3]. The conservative treatment is universally considered as the first line intervention, and the British National Institute for Health and Clinical Excellence (NICE) with the International Continence Society (ICS) recommend it as the first step [4–7]. As a matter of fact, a damaged pelvic floor can be improved through re-education exercises [9], and after them, approximately 65 % of women will improve, with 30–50 % ending up to surgery [8, 10, 11].

Principles of physiotherapy include a combination of different approaches:

- To teach how to overcome difficulties in movement using a combination of educational methods
- To stimulate sensory and motor pathways by encouraging normal movement patterns in order to normalize or restore the muscle and regain the motor control
- To improve muscle strength, endurance, and function through task-specific treatments, and restore normal motor function

All of the above points are intended to improve short- and long-term motivation and adherence to the health-enhancing behavior.

S. Minoli
UOC di Medicina Riabilitativa,
Centro di Riabilitazione "Villa Beretta" dell'Ospedale Valduce,
Costa Masnaga (Lc), Italy
e-mail: simonaminoli@libero.it

D. Riva, G. Minini (eds.), *Childbirth-Related Pelvic Floor Dysfunction: Risk Factors, Prevention, Evaluation, and Treatment*,
DOI 10.1007/978-3-319-18197-4_13

13.2 The Physiology

The pelvic floor is an interrelated system of organs, muscles, nerves, and connective tissue working synergistically as a dynamic system in balanced tension: its denervation, and the consequent muscle dysfunctions, can result in loss of the pelvic support organ, which can be followed by genital prolapse and urinary and/or fecal incontinence.

In order to plan the re-education program, the pelvic floor dysfunction should be analyzed on three levels of scientific background.

13.2.1 Motor Control

The central governance of the bladder provides a good example of the interplay network between the cortical motor system, the autonomic, and the somatic nervous system with the modulatory effects of the pudendal nerve. The functional magnetic resonance can identify the cerebral zones where bladder filling and voiding are regulated: reductions in the activation of the insula, of the right frontal operculum and of the anterior cingulate cortex suggest that treatment with EMG – biofeedback or pelvic floor muscle training (PFMT) or contraction-exercises [12–13] can change the emotional behavior related to micturition. The central nervous system coordinates and controls all the structures involved in opening and closing of urethra and anus as a switch mechanism. The anterior portion of the pubococcygeus muscle is a precise motor sensitive feedback zone that controls the tension in the vaginal membrane. Proportionate tensions are essential to maintain continence at rest because motor units of pelvic floor muscles are continuously activated (except during voiding or defecation), and their action increases with bladder or bowel activation. Defects, such as urinary stress incontinence and pelvic organ prolapse, have been associated with EMG alterations that may represent either loss of motor units or failure of central activation [14]. Recently, signs of dysfunction in the neural control (such as changes in the activation patterns) have been reported between the pubococcygeus [15], the levator ani, and the urethral sphincter [16].

Every sensory information from the pelvic region is relevant for the neural motor control of the pelvic floor muscles (PFM) and for the decision to activate the motor pattern. Lesions of fibers innervating the external anal sphincter are frequent (2–19 %) during childbirth and are caused either by spontaneous laceration or by episiotomy and can cause reduction in the contraction of the pubovisceral portion of the levator ani and in the external anal sphincter [17, 18].

13.2.2 Postural Balance

Posture is the result of multiple and complex processes that involve all the parts of the body and its relationship with the environment. The interactions among the different anatomic districts occur at different levels and are influenced by different starting conditions; alterations of imbalances produce a structural and physiological re-organization of the anatomic structures in order to improve the dynamic posture.

A good posture requires an orchestrate recruitment of the muscles of the whole system, which is limited by respiratory, pelvic, diaphragmatic, abdominal, and multifidus muscles. The peritoneum and perineum support comes from their connection to the pelvis and to the endopelvic fascia which is a unique network of connective tissue able to strength the muscle and its tendon insertions and to accommodate the viscera's cohabitation. It is well established that transversus abdominis plays a crucial role in optimal function of the lumbopelvic region; fascial tension is thought as the mechanism by which this muscle contributes to intersegmental and intrapelvic stiffness. Diastasis rectus abdominis (DRA) has the potential to disrupt this mechanism and is a common post-delivery occurrence [19].

13.2.3 Sphincter Capacity

Incontinence disorders, caused by pudendal nerve injuries, involve the urethral hypermotility, its external sphincter, the mucosal sealing effect, and the striated muscle activity. Urethra has three normal positions: resting closure, closure during effort and opening during micturition; and each state is the result of muscles forces whose contraction is required to open or close the sphincter. There are three directional muscle forces zone: *upper* (pubococcygeus and elevator plate) that stretches the organs forward or backward, *middle* (longitudinal muscle of the anus) which closes the bladder neck during effort and opens it during micturition and *lower* (perineal membrane) for stabilization of the distal parts of the urethra. Muscle's slow-twitch fibers maintain the urethral closure during effort, while the fast-twitch fibers are recruited to close the system further. After vaginal delivery, changes occur in muscle function: the urethral reaction, the simultaneous passive transmission of the abdominal pressure to the urethra and the "guarding reflex" are compromised and that is critical; furthermore, coughing increases the pelvic floor muscle's activity and induces an important decrease of the bladder neck's mobility, with its stabilization. "Squeezing" of the pelvic diaphragm is a movement explained only by the voluntary contraction of the puborectalis muscle and this is radically different from what is observed during coughing and straining. Levator ani, puborectalis, and anal sphincter muscles provide the majority of control for anal continence and they are constantly active. The puborectalis muscle works independently of the three directional forces, maintains the "anorectal" angle, facilitates continence, and has to be relaxed to allow defecation.

13.3 Clinical Pictures

Disorders that can be treated by physiotherapy:

- *Sensory–motor disorders or neuroaprassia is* the reduction of the sensitive perception and of the muscle activation (often on one side) due to the surface damage of the pudendal S2–S4 roots; alterations of muscle's morphology and asymmetric contractions can also be observed.

- *Micturition dysfunction* is generally related to laxity of the external urethral ligament and to disorders of the low urinary tract (LUT). These symptoms can be stress or urge incontinence, when coughing, straining, or even at rest; they can also be associated with altered emptying, voiding hesitancy, interrupted stream, raised residual urine volume, nicturia, and discomfort.
- *Postural disorders* are sensory–motor changes in pelvic, spinal, and respiratory functions related to biomechanical problems of the sacral and lumbar spine and of the muscle's area innervated by the S2–S4 roots. Trunk flexion, upper limb asymmetric or obturator internus, psoas, and piriformis shortening can be observed. Some muscles of the pelvic girdle may compensate for limitations of the pelvic floor in neutralizing the intra-abdominal pressure rises, by stiffening the sacroiliac joint, allowing backward rotation of the sacrum, and stabilizing the spine. Example of maladaptive movement patterns and poor stabilizing may be seen as abdominal bulging and breathing holding; excessive internal/external oblique activation with posterior pelvic tilt and flexor thoracolumbar attitude, excessive erector spinae activation with anterior pelvic tilt and thoracolumbar extension.
- *Anorectal dysfunction* is the inability to evacuate or to contain the rectal contents. It can be due to reduction of muscle thickness, loss of innervations, and motor disorders (of the levator plate, the longitudinal muscles, the anus, the puborectalis muscles, and the external anal sphincter).
- *Pelvic and perineal pain,* is due to laxity of the uterosacral ligaments and/or to spasm of the obturator muscle. It is a condition marked by dragging abdominal pain (often on one side), low sacral backache, aching or cramping pain in the vaginal and rectal area or in the coccyx and in the tailbone; symptoms can often be triggered or exacerbated by sitting, defecation, or by other motor activities stretching the pelvic floor. These symptoms are more frequent in case of dystocia or macrosomia. This picture, in the absence of neurological disease, is defined as overactive pelvic floor (OAPF) and is characterized by ischemic mucosa, sustained muscles contraction and forceful closure of the urethral sphincter.
- *Pudendal neuralgia* is defined as a neuropathic pain in one or more of the areas innervated by the pudendal nerve or by one of its branches: rectum, anus, urethra, perineum and the genital area (clitoris, mons pubis, vulva, lower third of the vagina, and labia).
- Typically, the perineal discomfort can evolve in chronic pelvic pain (CPP) which is not modified by standing or lying down, and can be exacerbated by sitting and is associated with sciatica and low back pain.
- *Sexual dysfunction* is lack of orgasm or feeling of "strange sensation" or loss of sexual desire. This condition is characterized by excessive activity of pubovisceral muscles that cause pain; the muscles become taut, short, and spasmodic with a modified activation pattern. These symptoms are often associated with the OAPF (overactive pelvic floor).

13.4 Rehabilitation Treatment

The rehabilitation course can develop a variety of interventions:

1. At first, program evaluates the pelvic floor situation (active straight, articular, neural, and visceral system tests), promotes continence, selects the correct aids, controls pain, and takes care of the perineal muscles. Some women will benefit simply from learning how to control their muscles; others will need an individualized approach, particularly if in the first assessment severe injuries of the pelvic floor has been observed. Rehabilitation program should assess the patients for posture, strength, flexibility, balance as well as for any other musculoskeletal structure involved. For women with incontinence of urine, stool, or flatus, the re-education program should be individually tailored. Key components of success include motivational strategies, to prevent embarrassment and information about anatomy, physiology, and dysfunction of the pelvic floor and of the lower tract urinary [20]. Before beginning the treatment, it is advisable to have a detailed bladder and bowel diary [21] to lead behavioral interventions and lifestyle changes. The diary must provide information on type of voiding dysfunction, bowel habit, fluid intake, time and volume of micturition, time of each incontinent episode, and circumstances or reasons for dribbling urine. The bladder retraining is a form of behavioral therapy and its aim is to help regain the bladder control by increasing its capacity and thereby reducing the symptoms. Keeping a record of a frequency/volume chart, and urine volume/liquid intake plays a central role in bladder training, because the patient is asked to increase the intervals between voiding, which results in a gradual increase in bladder capacity, and the diary is used to monitor the treatment success. The addition of pelvic floor therapeutic exercises is beneficial. Re-education program goes on with an accurate transvaginal assessment of pelvic floor muscle zone, to determine abnormalities, overactivity or underactivity, lack of coordination, reduction of sensitivity, tenderness, and pain or hyperalgesia. This later is a common symptom that can be treated with interventions such as support garments, clothing considerations for abdominal support, review use of heat/ice or diatermia, transcutaneous electrical nerve stimulation (TENS), and kinesiotaping applications for abdominal wall weakness. The pelvic floor motor function such as the resting tone, the contraction strength, the reflex response to cough or to Valsalva maneuver can be altered. The PERFECT scheme (pressure, endurance, repetitions, every contraction time) and a dynamic evaluation (on standing position, at rest, and during exercise) can be helpful. The examination of the puborectalis and the external anal sphincter can be performed in left lateral position, at rest, and during squeezing.
2. The re-education process starts with the therapeutic exercises. Their rational is to re-program a coordinated behavior pattern consisting of the following:
   - Coordination between the PFMs and the external urethral sphincter (SUE) relaxation at the start of voiding and during the bladder empting.

- A good PFM function during episodes of detrusor overactivity.
- A voluntary contraction of PFM to hit the target: high bladder compliance versus micturition control.
- A voluntary activation able to control a maximally filled bladder or liquid stool-filled rectal ampulla during additional physical stress, coughing, sneezing, deep breathing, walking, and so on.

  At the beginning of the program we often have to stimulate voluntary contractions because patients may have different, inefficient responses as "fasciculation" or slow activation or weak asymmetric contractions or "no response at all."

  In the last case, we can use neuromuscular facilitation (stretch reflex), augmented proprioceptive sensory inputs, and motor control exercises, performed in lying position. We can also electrically stimulate the large diameter nerves supplying the pelvic floor and the urethral striated muscles and that induces skeletal muscles training, remodels smooth muscle and connective tissues and modulates bladder, bowel and sexual function [22]. The depolarization of the pudendal nerve also generates a reflex response with the inhibition of the overactive sphincter: re-organization, re-coordination and awareness of the lower urinary tract are the effects. In case of "overactive bladder," muscle electrical stimulation (EMS) rebalances the descending excitatory information by artificially activating bladder-inhibitors reflex. This strategy is adjunctive to voluntary exercise and to anticholinergic drugs in increasing the strength of a weak PFM, reducing voiding frequency, and increasing the voided volume. Way of application, stimulation site, electrical parameters, protocol, and equipment characteristics can be adapted to the single clinical case. Another common motor learning strategy, used to train patients to improve the control of the muscle recruitment, is the biofeedback technique. This process can be performed with different strategies such as EMG/mmHg catheter, probe surface monitoring, perineal and abdominal ultrasound, vaginal retention sensation, and cystourethroscopy.

3. When the pelvic floor muscle assessment is equal to 2 (Perfect scheme), exercises goes on with a training program that must satisfy three principles: overload (applied to strength, endurance, and function/technique), specificity (exercise's objective/functional task) and reversibility (loss of hypertrophy). In the 1st week, the strength increase is mediated by the neuromuscular adaptations to conditioning. Training starts with exercises of low-level control, on lying position and with empty bladder, and then continues with progressive filling, to perform several maximum contractions of shorter duration, with a minimal rest period, to realize the fast-twitch fibers' recruitment [23, 24]. The physiotherapist can help the patient to improve the bladder control, at first voiding desire, teaching how to activate muscles to suppress detrusor contractions: stop, stay still, squeeze PFM quickly three to five times (repeat as needed), wait, take deep breaths, and so on. For this cognitive process [25], any form of feedback seems an appropriate learning strategy: manual examination can be used during

dynamic functions such as during exercising, lying, and standing. Only when the pelvic floor muscle assessment is equal to 3 (Perfect scheme), the use of vaginal cones exercise [26] can be better, on standing, walking, or on treadmill. Biofeedback technique assisted during pelvic floor exercising can be used.

The physiotherapist can help the patient in changing the motor pattern's recruitment and assist her to modify physical activities during daily bladder monitoring. The training must identify the motor activities that seem to trigger incontinence and realize motor coordination during change in posture. On sitting position, for example, the patient can learn how to balance unsupported sitting postures where greater pelvic floor muscle activity [27] is required. The control of the sphincter, on standing position, and of the puborectalis (PR) muscle activity during intra-abdominal pressure increase (as cough or sneeze or deep breath) is important because the increase of the closure pressure is differently transmitted to the urethral length. Such voluntary motor control can be realized with postural alignment and exercises that balance and stabilize the trunk, the spine, and the upper limbs; later also by walking and running. It is recommended to wait until the patient is continent before starting water aerobic fitness works.

The aim of this education program is to learn the "habit to control" during the everyday life; such a skill is possible only by regeneration and new planning of the motor and neuronal pathways.

4. Anorectal exercise training

Many patients after vaginal delivery need to be helped also for problems related to bowel disorders, evacuations difficulties [28] or anal incontinence [29]. In clinical practice, it makes sense to combine anterior and posterior perineal zone approaches in re-training program to maximize benefits. Patients can benefit from education on physiological bowel management, evacuation training, correct posture, breathing, pushing, muscle relaxing with defecation, avoiding laxatives, observing a proper diet, assuming fluids and practicing physical activity. It is worth noting that therapeutic exercises, postural adjustments, and some procedures (as feedback) can improve the muscle control on external anal sphincter (EAS) and PR recruitment. In case of *anal sphincter overactivity,* abnormal increase tension, and muscle retraction, the treatment includes a coccyx's mobilization, muscle stretching of EAS and PR, and postural control exercises to relax, or EMS with analgesia parameters to control pain. On *paradoxical contraction* during defecation, exercise can teach how to control the altered activation pattern between SAE and PR muscles. In case of dissociated activation pattern, manometry, or EMG anal probe or surface electrodes biofeedback are used to enhance the rectal sensitivity to distension. In the gastroenterology setting, "biofeedback" is often quoted as the management of first choice for *anal incontinence* [30, 31] because it can improve the closure pressure dependent to alter recruitment of the EAS. When there is low muscle activity, it has been postulated that electrical stimulation may increase muscle hypertrophy and neuroplastic changes and increase the representation of the anorectum. In case of anal incontinence, using a rectal balloon, the patient can learn how to resist to the urge to defecate by squeezing the anal sphincter in order to resist to the drop of the anal pressure that follows the rectal distension (the rectoanal inhibitor reflex).

When pelvic floor disorders do not respond to physiotherapy, surgical intervention or sacral nerve stimulation can be suggested but there are insufficient reliable data to make a positive recommendation for one technique over another.

Physiotherapists have to be guided by the patient's choices and characteristics and the treatment should address all factors that may interact with the pelvic floor muscle disorders. Much remains to be learnt about pelvic floor disorders. It is hoped that progresses in understanding the underlying mechanism will lead to further advances in organ-specific therapy.

References

1. MacLennan AH, Taylor AW, Wilson DH (2000) The prevalence of pelvic floor disorders and their relationship to gender, parity and mode of delivery. BJOG 107:1460–1470
2. UustalFornell E, Wingren G, Kjolhede P (2004) Factors associated with pelvic floor dysfunction with emphasis on urinary and fecal incontinence and genital prolapse: an epidemiological study. Acta Obstet Gynecol Scand 83:383–389
3. Fitz FF, Costa TF, Yamamoto DM, Resende AP, Stupp L, Sartori MG, Girao MJ, Castro RA (2012) Impact of pelvic floor muscle training on quality of life in women with urinary incontinence. Rev Assoc Med Bras 58(2):155–159
4. Morkved S, Bo K (2014) Pelvic floor muscle training after childbirth can prevent and treat urinary incontinence. A supervised training protocol following strength-training principles, emphazising close to maximum contractions and lasting at least 8 weeks is recommended. PFMT should be incorpored as a routine part of women's exercise programs in general. 2013 Systematic Review. Br J Sports Med 48(4):299–310
5. Consensus conference. Urinary incontinence in adults (1989) JAMA. 261:2685–2690.
6. Fantl JA, Newman DK, Colling J (1996) Urinary incontinence guideline panel. Urinary incontinence in adults: acute and chronic management. Clinical practice guideline. No.2 1996 update AHCPR Publication No.96-0682 6(3):19–24. Rockville: Agency for Health Care Policy and Research, Public Health Service, US Department of Health and Human Services
7. Abrams P, Cardozo L, Wein A, Khoury S (2009) Conservative management is the main approach to UI in men at the primary care level, and is often considered to be simple and low cost. The term 'conservative management' describes any treatment that does not involve pharmacological or surgical intervention. However, for conditions, such as OAB, conservative strategies are often combined with drug treatment. 4° International Consultation on Incontinence Paris, pp 5–8
8. Labrie J, van der Graaf Y, Buskens E, Tiersma SE, van der Vaart HC (2009) Protocol for physiotherapy Or TVT Randomized Efficacy Trial (PORTRET): a multicenter randomized controlled trial to assess the cost-effectiveness of the tension vaginal tape versus pelvic floor muscle training in women with symptomatic moderate to severe urinary incontinence. BMC Womens Health 9:24
9. Carneiro EF, Araujo Ndos S, Beuttenmull L, Vieiria PC, Cader SA (2010) The anatomical-functional characteristics of the pelvic floor and quality of life of women with urinary incontinence subjected to perineal exercises. Actas Urol Esp 35(9):788–793
10. Dumoulin C, Martin C, Elliott V (2013) Randomized control trial of physiotherapy for post partum stress incontinence:7.years follow-up. Neurourol Urodyn 32(5):449–454
11. Ahlund S, Nordgen B, Wilander EL (2013) Is home-based pelvic floor muscle training effective in treatment of urinary incontinence after birth in primiparous women? A randomized controlled trial. Acta Obstet Gynecol Scand 92(8):909–915

12. Stasa D, Derek G, Werner S, Cathy C, Neil M (2009) Brain activity measured by functional magnetic resonance imaging is related to patient reported urgency incontinence severity. J Urol 08(155)
13. Di Gangi Herms AM, Veit R, Reiseenauer C (2006) Functional imaging of stress urinary incontinence. Neuroimage 29:267–275, 200
14. Cundiff G, Addison A (1998) Management of pelvic prolapse. Obstet Gynecol Clin N America 25(4):90:19–26
15. Salvioli B, Bharucha AE, Rath-Harvey D (2001) Rectal compliance capacity, and rectoanal sensation in fecal incontinence. Am J Gastroenterol 96(7):2158–2168
16. Cescon C, Raimondi E, Merletti R (2014) Characterization of the motor units of the external anal sphincter in pregnant women with multichannel surface EMG. Int Urogynecol J 25:1097–1103
17. Enck P, Franz H, Azpiroz F, Fernandez-Fraga X, Hinninghofen H, Kaske-Bretag K, Bottin A, Martina S, Merletti R (2004) Innervation zone of the external anal sphincter in healthy male and female subjects. Digestion 69:123–130
18. Cescon C, Riva D, Zacesta V, Drusany Staric K, Martsidis K, Protsepko O, Baessler K, Merletti R (2014) Effect of vaginal delivery on the external anal sphincter muscle innervation pattern evaluated by multichannel surface EMG: results of the multicentre study TASI-2. Int Urogynecol J 25:1491–1499
19. Spitznagle TM, Leong FC, van Dillen LR (2007) Prevalence of diastasis recti abdominis in a urogynecological patient population. Int Urogynecol J 18(3):321–8
20. Munariz R, Kim NN, Goldstein I et al (2002) Biology of female sexual function. Urol Clin North Am 29:685–693
21. Laycock J, Standley A, Crothers E (2001) Patient education and management. In: Clinical guidelines for the physiotherapy management of females aged 16 to 65 years with stress urinary incontinence. Chartered Society of Physiotherapy, London, p 19
22. Locher JL, Roth DL, Goode PS (2001) Reliability assessment of the bladder diary for urinary incontinence in older women. J Gerontol A Biol Sci Med Sci 56:M32–M35
23. Petros PP, Skilling PM (2001) Pelvic floor rehabilitation in the female according to the integral theory of female urinary incontinence. First report. Eur J Obstet Gynecol Reprod Biol 94:264–269
24. McNevin N, Gabriele W, Carlson C (2000) Effects of attentional focus, self control and dyad training on motor learning: implications for physical rehabilitation. Phys Ther 80(4):373–385
25. Bourcier AP, Burgio KL (2004) Biofeedback therapy. In: Bourcier AP, McGuire EJ, Abrams P (eds) Pelvic floor disorders. Sauders-Elsevier, Philadelphia, pp 297–311
26. Hobday DI, Aziz Q, Thacker N (2001) A study of the cortical processing of ano-rectal sensation using functional MRI. Brain 124:361–368
27. Jones R, Comerford M, Sapford R (2002) Pelvic floor stability and trunk muscle co-activation. In: Layock J, Haslam J (eds) Therapeutic management of incontinence and pelvic pain. Springer, London, pp 66–71
28. Sapsford RR, Richardson CA, Stanton WR (2006) Sitting posture affects pelvic floor muscle activity in parous woman: an observational study. Aust J Physiother 52:219–222
29. Bleijenberg G, Kujipers HC (1987) Treatment of the spastic pelvic floor syndrome with biofeedback. Dis Colon Rectum 50(2):108–111
30. Whitehead WE, Wald A, Norton N (2001) Treatment options for fecal incontinence: consensus conference report. Dis Colon Rectum 44:131–144
31. Hosker G, Norton C, Brazzelli M (2002) Electrical stimulation for fecal incontinence in adults. Cochrane Database Syst Rev 2007(3):CD001310

Surgery for Urinary Incontinence and Prolapse Shortly After Childbirth

14

Luisa Ricci

14.1 Prolapse Surgery After Pregnancy

Onset of pelvic organ prolapse (POP) in postpartum period is a well-noted disease among young women. Pregnancy itself, hormonal modification during gestation and baby passage through the birth canal determine a mechanical distortion that damages connective tissues, vessels, nerves, and muscular structures [1, 2]. Morbidity of pelvic organ prolapse has an impact on social, psychological, and sexual well-being.

Modification in pelvic organ support may be permanent or transitory. Generally, women are examined 6–8 weeks postpartum: during that time the reproductive tract, as well as the whole body, is believed to return to the original aspect. Chen et al. [3] demonstrated that the process of reconstruction is not completed until 1-year postpartum: Connective tissues and pelvic floor contractility takes up to 6 months to recovery after parturition.

Stage II prolapse is a common finding in postpartum women, with a prevalence of about 50 % 6 weeks after birth, and of 30 % 6 months postpartum, as well as in those presenting for general gynecological care [4]. Although the definition of anatomic prolapse has been defined by the National Institutes of Health [5] as descent of stage I or greater, perhaps the definition of "normal" should be reconsidered. The threshold at which pathology occurs, what is defined as symptomatic prolapse, and the optimal time of intervention, still remains unclear. There are no guidelines about the management of patients with vaginal prolapse immediately after pregnancy. Symptomatic women, which need surgical approach, are a little percentage of the total. Only symptomatic patients with POP-Q > stage 2 are candidate to the operating theater. There is no clear difference between surgery after childbirth or in older

L. Ricci
Department of Obstetric and Gunecologic, Ospedale Montecchio E. (RE), Italy
e-mail: luisa.ricci@me.com

D. Riva, G. Minini (eds.), *Childbirth-Related Pelvic Floor Dysfunction: Risk Factors, Prevention, Evaluation, and Treatment*,
DOI 10.1007/978-3-319-18197-4_14

ages, but especially in younger women, when surgery is necessary, a careful counselling is mandatory. Great part of people think that a surgical reconstruction of genital prolapse will restore completely not only the pelvic floor anatomy, but also the pelvic function. As a result of a surgical procedure, patients must be informed about effect of scarring, fibrosis, weakened or reduced elasticity of the vaginal wall as well as impaired nerve function [6, 7].

The first question is about the best surgical approach. If the anatomical defect is in the anterior compartment (cystocele) or in the posterior one (rectocele), vaginal route is the better choice. More than 80 % of surgical repair involves anterior vaginal wall, with recurrence rate, following traditional native tissues repair, which varies from 30 to 60 %. Implementation in surgical techniques, with a proper dissection of the pubo-vesico-cervical fascia or a site-specific repair, and a close knowledge about the pathophysiology of POP, lead to a better anatomical result and to an improvement in quality of life. Those consideration reinforce the concept that native tissue repair is the first choice in young women. If rectocele is present, an accurate evaluation of rectal function must precede any surgical approach: bowel symptoms or difficult defecation leads patient to use manual pressure to defecate. Wexner's Continence Grading Scale, transanal ultrasound and manometry are unavoidable in correct evaluation of this vaginal segment. Good anatomical and subjective cure rates are reached with posterior colporrhaphy and site-specific repair. There is no place for mesh augmentation because of high rate of dyspareunia, exposure, and worsening of bowel function.

After FDA pronunciation in 2011 [8], transvaginal mesh repair is not indicated in young women and in first surgery. Mesh insertion results in higher rates of adverse effect including mesh exposure, buttock and pelvic pain or discomfort, and de novo incontinence. Women must be informed about risk of recurrence both in the same compartment such as in the unrepaired site, because of a variation in the vaginal axis. In spite of an improvement in anatomic outcome, the reoperation rate is increased in comparison with a native tissues repair [9].

Symptomatic hysterocele needs a detailed evaluation to reveal cases of cervical elongation. In this group of patients, if patients desire a uterine-sparing procedure, a sacrospinous hysteropexy would not give a good anatomical result. Manchester procedure [10] is a practice specifically performed in patients with symptomatic genital prolapse in combination with cervical elongation. Women must be informed about elevated risk of cervical incompetence or cervical stenosis leading to mechanical dysmenorrhea, secondary infertility, or hematometra. In well-selected cases, Manchester procedure restores good apical support and vaginal length and maintains the physiological vaginal axis.

In premenopausal women, who have completed their family program, vaginal hysterectomy is the first choice: This procedure, added to a plication of uterosacral ligaments, represents an efficient treatment for symptomatic POP, and has been demonstrated to be less invasive in terms of hospital stay, blood loss, and return to daily activity [11–13].

For women who have not completed their family, or longing for uterine sparing surgery, sacrospinous cervicocolpopexy must be considered. Menstrual disorders, uterine or cervical pathology, and endometrial hyperplasia are absolute or relative contraindication to this procedure. In 1989, Richardson et al. [14] reported a case series of five women with utero-vaginal prolapse, age between 24 and 31 years, having a transvaginal sacrospinous hysteropexy. No recurrences were observed during a follow-up period of 6–24 month. SSH is a safe and effective alternative to hysterectomy in treating uterovaginal prolapse. SSH in associated with shorter operation time, less blood loss, shorter hospitalization, and earlier recovery and return to daily activities [15, 16].

14.2 Sexual Function and Pain After POP Surgery

Pelvic organ prolapse has a negative impact on sexual function: Vaginal bulging, pelvic pain, diminished sensibility are the most frequently reported issues [17]. Up to 64 % of sexually active women with POP suffer from sexual dysfunction [18]. Physicians are often inadequately trained to approach this problem, so it remains underestimated. Anne-Marie Roos et al. [19] demonstrated that both urinary incontinence (UI) and POP affect the sexual life of women. All stages of sexual excitement are affected by the fear for coital incontinence. Instead women with POP have a worse genital image than women who have never been diagnosed with prolapse. Zielinskj et al. [20] have shown that genital body image and sexual health are related, especially in the light of sexual satisfaction and desire. The most referred topics, affecting sexual satisfaction, are decreasing sexual desire, less lubrication, dyspareunia, fear of urinary or anal incontinence (especially gas incontinence).

In literature, there are few studies about sexual function after POP surgery and cases evaluated are not enough to have statistical significance. Women who had POP surgery with native tissues generally report improvement in sexual function for cessation of incontinence and sexual function. Pelvic pain and dyspareunia after prolapse repair are often multifactorial in nature, with vaginal shortening and narrowing, ipoestrogenism, and dryness playing a significant role [21]. It is also well accepted that the rate of dyspareunia, especially after a posterior compartment surgery, may approach 40 %. Lower vaginal wall sensibility is associated with vaginal POP surgery and/or suburetral sling procedure, but does not correlate with vaginal dryness and anorgasmia. Low rates of post-surgical sexual symptoms might be due to an improvement of the patients' confidence and body image because of correction of the anatomical defect and cure of the associated symptoms such as urinary incontinence and bulging. Diminished sexual function after surgery can be the result of scarring, fibrosis, short or narrow vagina, contracted pelvic floor, weakened or reduced elasticity of the vagina as well as impaired nerve function [22–24].

14.3 Pregnancy and Birth After POP Surgery

Looking to the literature we can find a great number of uterine-sparing repairs, but very little is published about subsequent pregnancy, way of birth, and long-term follow-up [25, 26].

When a systematic review about pregnancy after prolapse surgery is performed, it is possible to find only few case reports and case series. There is no information available regarding the incidence of childbirth following pelvic procedures and no data about incidence of repeated POP surgery following delivery. Too little is known for a complete counselling about safety of pregnancy and mode of delivery after such surgery and the impact of further pregnancy on the outcome of the original procedure. Case reports generally suggest a scheduled cesarean section as the preferred mode of delivery after Prolapse surgery. In case of transvaginal sling instead little more data are available [27–29]. In case series vaginal delivery is referred as safe, and no higher recurrence is demonstrated. Anyway a second sling placement is considered safer than a scheduled cesarean section.

Given the relative rarity of pregnancy following any pelvic floor repair procedure, it is difficult to formulate any recommendation and studies are limited because of small numbers and their retrospective nature.

14.4 Incontinence Surgery After Pregnancy

Urinary incontinence affects about 25 % of women, and stress incontinence is the most common type, with a prevalence of 50 % [30]. Pregnancy is an important risk factor for urinary incontinence: the onset of urinary incontinence during pregnancy is a negative prognostic factor for persistence in the postpartum period and later in life. About 20 % of pregnant women reports urge incontinence, but the most common type of urinary symptom during pregnancy is stress urinary incontinence, with a prevalence of about 40 % [31]. Since pelvic support may be disrupted during pregnancy and after delivery, most physicians recommend delaying surgery until women have completed their family planning. Conservative therapy and pelvic muscle rehabilitation is the first line treatment [32–34], while surgical correction is indicated when conservative treatment fails and it commonly consists in transobturator sling or single incision slings. Low complication rate and good rates of success associated with such procedures give reason of increasing number of women requiring surgical resolution of stress incontinence, also in younger ages [35]. Although a number of reports in the literature describe pregnancy successfully completed by vaginal delivery and cesarean section, there is no consensus about the preferred mode of delivery [27, 36]. Pregnancy itself represent a risk factor for recurrence of stress incontinence in women treated with suburetral sling, because of level of progestogen, increase of uterine size and weight applied on the suspensory structures. In many studies rate of recurrence after vaginal delivery is reported to be higher than after cesarean section, but no statistical significance is achieved. If stress incontinence does not recur during pregnancy, a vaginal delivery is safe and does not increase the risk of severe or permanent stress incontinence [28, 29]. In case of recurrence surgical options are bulking agents or a second sling procedure.

References

1. Lukacz ES, Lawrence JM, Contreras R, Nager CW, Luber KM (2006) Parity, mode of delivery and pelvic floor disorders. Obstet Gynecol 107:1253–1260
2. Leijonhufvud A, Lundholm C, Nattingius S, Granath F, Andolf E, Altman D (2011) Risks of stress urinary incontinence and pelvic organ prolapse surgery in relation to mode of childbirth. Am J Obstet Gynecol 204:70–74
3. Chen Y, Li F-Y, Lin X, Chen J, Chen C, Guess MK (2013) The recovery of pelvic organ support during the first year postpartum. BJOG 120:1430–1437
4. Wai CY, McIntire DD, Atnip SD, Schaffer JI, Bloom SL, Leveno KJ (2011) Urodynamic indices and pelvic organ prolapse quantification 3 month after vaginal delivery in primiparous women. Int Urogynecol J 22:1293–1298
5. Weber AM, Abrams P, Brubaker L, Cundiff G, Davis G, Dmochowski RR et al (2011) The standardization of terminology for researchers in female pelvic floor disorders. Int Urogynecol J Pelvic Floor Dysfunct 12:178–186
6. Paraiso MF, Barber MD, Muir TW, Walters MD (2006) Rectocele repair: a randomized trial of three surgical techniques including graft augmentation. Am J Obstet Gynecol 195: 1762–1771
7. Grimes CL, Tan-Kim J, Whitcomb EL, Lukacz ES, Menefee SA (2012) Long-term outcomes after native tissue vs biological graft augmented repair in the posterior compartment. Int Urogynecol J 23:597–604
8. Food and Drug Administration (2011) FDA Safety Communication: update on seroìious complications associated with transvaginal placement of surgical mesh for pelvic organ prolapse. http://www.fda.gov/MedicalDevices/Safety/AlertandNotices/umc262435.htm
9. Gomelsky A, Penson DF, Dmochowski RR (2011) Pelvic organ prolapse (POP) surgery: the evidence for the repairs. BJU Int 107:1704–1719
10. Ayhan A, Esin S, Guven S, Salman C, Ozyuncu O (2006) The Manchester operation for uterine prolapse. Int J Gynecol Obstet 92(3):228–233
11. Salvatore S, Athanasiou S, Digesu GA, Soligo M, Sotiropoulou M, Serati M, Antsaklis A, Milani R (2009) Identification of risk factors for genital prolapse recurrence. Neurourol Urodyn 28:301–304
12. Pakbaz M, Mogren I, Lofgren M (2009) Outcomes of vaginal hysterectomy for uterovaginal prolapse: a population-based, retrospective, cross-sectional study of patient perceptions of results including sexual activity, urinary symptoms, and provided care. BMC Womens Health 9:9
13. Abdel-Fattah M, Familusi A, Fielding S, Ford J, Bhattacharya S (2011) Primary and repeat surgical treatment for female pelvic organ prolapse and incontinence in parous womenin the UK: a register linkage study. BMJ Open 1(2):e000206
14. Richardson DA, Scotti RJ, Ostergard DR (1989) Surgical management of uterine prolapse in young women. J Reprod Med 34:388–392
15. Dietz V, Van der Vaart CH, Van der Graaf Y, Heintz P, Schraffordt Koops S (2010) One-year follow-up after sacrospinous hysteropexy and vaginal hysterectomy for uterine descent: a randomized study. Int Urogynecol J 21:209–216
16. Feiner B, Gietelink L, Maher C (2010) Anterior vaginal mesh sacrospinous hysteropexy and posterior fascial plication for anterior compartement dominated uterovaginal prolapse. Int Urogynecol J 21:203–208
17. Lakeman M, van der Vaart H, Laan E, Roovers JP (2011) The effect of prolapse surgery on vaginal sensibility. J Sex Med 8:1239–1245
18. Glavind K, Larsen T, Lindquist AS (2015) Sexual function in women before and after surgery for pelvic organ prolapse. Acta Obstet Gynecol Scand 94(1):80–85
19. Roos AM, Thakar R, Siltan AH, Burger CW, Paulus ATG (2014) Pelvic floor dysfunction: women's sexual concerns unrevealed. J Sex Med 11:743–752

20. Zielinski R, Miller J, Low LK, Sampselle C, DeLancey JOL (2012) The relationship between pelvic organ prolapse, genital body image, and sexual health. Neurourol Urodynam 31: 1145–1148
21. Pauls RN, Andre Silva W, Rooney CM, Siddighi S, Kleeman SD, Dryfhout V, Karram MM (2007) Sexual function after vaginal surgery for pelvic organ prolapse and urinary incontinence. Am J Obstet Gynecol 197:622.e1–7
22. Dalpiaz O, Kerschbaumer A, Mitterberger M, Pinggera GM, Colleselli D, Bartsch G, Strasser H (2008) Female sexual dysfunction: a new urogynaecological research field. BJU Int 101:717–721
23. Kavvadias T, Baessler K, Schuessler B (2012) Pelvic pain in urogynecology. PartII: treatment options in patients with lower urinary tract symptoms. Int Urogynecol J 23:553–561
24. Edenfield AL, Levin PJ, Dieter AA, Amundsen CL, Siddiqui NY (2015) Sexual activity and vaginal topography in women with symptomatic pelvic floor disorders. J Sex Med 12: 416–423
25. Lewis CM, Culligan P (2011) Sacrohisteropexy followed by successful pregnancy and eventual reoperation for prolapse. Int Urogynecol J 23:957–959
26. Kuntepe Y, Cetinkaya K, Karasu Y (2013) Pregnancy and delivery after anterior vaginal mesh replacement: a case presentation. Int Urogynecol J 24:345–347
27. Huser M, Belkov IA, Janku P, Sedlakova K (2012) Pregnancy and delivery following midurethrale sling surgery for stress urinary incontinence. Int J Gynecol Obstet 119:117–120
28. Cavkaytar S, Kokanali MK, Ozer I, Erkilinc S, Aksakal OS, Doganay M (2015) Effect of pregnancy and delivery on urinary incontinence after the midurethral sling procedure. Int Urogynecol J 26(5):693–698
29. Tan HJ, Siu W, Faerber GJ, McGuire EJ, Latini JM (2010) Long-term durability of pubovaginal fascial slings in women who then become pregnant and deliver. Int Urogynecol J 21: 631–635
30. Hannestad YS, Rortveit G, Sandvik H, Hunskaar S (2000) Epidemiology of incontinence in the coutry of nord-trondelag. A community-based epidemiological survey of female urinary incontinence: the Norvegian EPICONT study. J Clin Epidemiol 53:1150–1157
31. Schytt E, Lindmark G, Waldenstrom U (2004) Symptoms of stress incontinence 1 year after childbirth: prevalence and predictors in a national Swedish sample. Acta Osbstet Gynecol Scand 83:928–936
32. Fritel X, Fauconnier A, Bader G (2010) Diagnosis and management of adult female stress urinary incontinence: guidelines for clinical practice from the French College of Gynaecologists and Obstetricians. Eur J Obstet Gynecol Reprod Biol 151:14–19
33. Sampselle CM, Miller JM, Mims BL, Delancey JOC, Ashton-Miller JA, Antonakos CL (1998) Effect of pelvic muscle exercise on transient incontinence during pregnancy and after birth. Obstet Gynecol 91(3):406–412
34. Morkoved S, Bo K, Schei B, Salvesen KA (2003) Pelvic floor muscle training during pregnancy to prevent urinary incontinence: a single blind randomized controlled trial. Obstet Gynecol 101(2):313–319
35. Nilsson CG, Palva K, Rezapour M, Falconer C (2008) Eleven years prospective follow-up of the tension-free vaginal tape procedure for then treatment of stress urinary incontinence. Int Urogynecol J 19:1043–1047
36. Tommaselli GA, Di Carlo C, Formisano C, Fabozzi A, Nappi C (2012) Vaginal delivery following single incision sling (TVT-Secur) for female stress urinary incontinence. J Obstet Gynaecol Res 39:608–610

A Practical Approach to Pelvic Floor Dysfunctions After Childbirth: Diagnostic and Therapeutic Flowcharts

15

Antonella Biroli

15.1 What Pelvic Floor Dysfunctions After Childbirth Should Be Considered?

Pregnancy and childbirth are well-known risk factors for pelvic dysfunction. Great attention was paid in the later years to urinary incontinence, as many women report this distressing condition in the first year after delivery. So, many studies were published in the attempt of correlating urinary incontinence with risk factors either inherent maternal or fetal or delivery factors. Despite its frequency, urinary incontinence is not the only possible unwished consequence of delivery. Other dysfunctions can affect women, but they are often less investigated by professionals and reported by women. Minor prevalence, or greater shame in complaining of these other symptoms, and moreover no knowledge about available treatment could account for this disparity of approach.

Urinary incontinence (UI) is reported by 10–38 % of women after delivery [1, 2], affecting 21 % of women during the 3 months postpartum according to an Italian study [3]. It is commonly accepted on the basis of data from literature and from clinical experience that prevalence decreases along the first year after delivery, but some longitudinal studies within the first year postpartum show small changes in prevalence over time [2, 4]. Stress incontinence is the most reported complaint, but urge or mixed incontinence are common too [1].

Anal incontinence (AI) is not an uncommon symptom in postpartum mothers, even more distressing than urinary incontinence. Women sometimes deem UI "a normal consequence of delivery," at least in the first year after delivery, but AI is never considered "normal." The reported prevalence of AI during postpartum varies markedly depending on the definitions of incontinence (anal or fecal), the

A. Biroli
Neurologic and Autonomic Dysfunctions Rehabilitation Unit,
San Giovanni Bosco Hospital, Turin, Italy
e-mail: biran@virgilio.it

D. Riva, G. Minini (eds.), *Childbirth-Related Pelvic Floor Dysfunction: Risk Factors, Prevention, Evaluation, and Treatment*,
DOI 10.1007/978-3-319-18197-4_15

evaluation tools, the elapsed time from delivery. Fecal incontinence affects 3–10 % of women after delivery and it seems to be less frequent at 1 year than in the first 6 months after delivery. Flatus incontinence is even more common, being reported by 6–49 % of women [1, 5–7]. Moreover, many women complain of distressing fecal urgency even if not really incontinent.

Pelvic organ prolapse (POP) can occur as a consequence of hormonal and mechanical changes during pregnancy and damage of pelvic floor connective and muscular supportive structures at delivery. Unfortunately, most studies evaluating the pelvic floor focus on the impact of delivery on urinary or anal incontinence with less attention to pelvic floor support. Unlike urinary incontinence, its diagnosis is problematic: there are often discrepancies between the "objective" measurement of descent of the vaginal walls or apex and prolapse symptoms [8]. Nevertheless, the few available data show that prolapse affects 83–100 % of women 5–22 weeks after delivery, being POPQ stage II at the examination in 35–52 % [9, 10]. After delivery the likelihood of finding a POPQ stage II prolapse declines during the first year postpartum [11], being 31 % at 6–12 months after delivery [12].

Dyspareunia after childbirth is probably related to mechanical, hormonal, and psychosexual factors but there is limited knowledge about it. According to the few studies that investigated dyspareunia during postpartum, it seems to be very common, affecting 17–44 % of the women at 6 months and 8–33 % of women at 12 months postpartum and being severe in one-third of them [13–15]. No link was found between dyspareunia and pelvic floor function (tone and strength) but we have no data about the link with other findings (e.g., scars, trigger points, vaginismus, and perineal stretching pain) that could account for a physical therapy approach.

Changes occur in *pelvic floor muscles* after delivery. Using magnetic resonance it is possible to show changes in muscle signal intensities, thickness, urogenital and levator hiatus areas, and perineal body position, and data suggest that connective tissue and pelvic floor muscle contractility can take up to 6 months to recover after parturition [16]. The muscle strength of the pelvic floor is reduced after vaginal birth but seems to return to the antepartum value 6–10 weeks postpartum in most women [17].

15.2 Are Treatments for Pelvic Floor Dysfunctions After Child Birth Available and Effective?

Conservative treatment, consisting of lifestyle interventions and rehabilitation, is a well-established approach for pelvic floor dysfunctions in general population.

To date the great majority of studies concerns urinary incontinence and there is consistent level I evidence, grade A recommendation, that pelvic floor muscle training is effective in the treatment of female urinary incontinence [18]. Nevertheless, a rehabilitative approach has also been proposed for treatment of POP, anal incontinence, pain, and dyspareunia.

Compared to urinary incontinence, studies about rehabilitation in pelvic floor dysfunctions other than urinary incontinence are fewer; nevertheless, several randomized controlled trials have shown that pelvic floor muscle training is effective in improving POP symptoms and/or severity in middle-aged women [19, 20]. A systematic review concluded that there is level 1, grade A evidence to recommend

PFMT in treatment of POP. One RCT found also that PFMT significantly improved PFM strength and thickness and narrowed the hiatus area in women with POP [19].

According to a recent review, rehabilitation could also be an effective treatment for fecal incontinence but despite the great number of studies in this field, in most cases they are uncontrolled trials or low-quality RCTs [18]. Moreover, biofeedback is widely used in the treatment of anal incontinence, so most studies concern the efficacy of rehabilitation when employing manometric biofeedback. The review concludes that pelvic floor muscle exercise is recommended as an early intervention in the treatment of fecal incontinence on the basis of low cost and morbidity, although there is little evidence of efficacy, and the add of biofeedback is recommended in case of inadequate relief of symptoms, given the numerous positive outcomes from uncontrolled trials (grade B recommendation). A Cochrane review concludes that there is only a suggestion for biofeedback and sphincter exercise effectiveness [21].

Evidences for effectiveness of rehabilitation in dyspareunia are poor. A few studies investigated the role of physical therapy in order to reduce pelvic floor hypertonia and vaginismus in vulvar pain syndromes causing dyspareunia, showing pain reduction in 50–70 % of women [22–24]. There is a need to conduct further RCTs to determinate whether physical therapy can be effective in dyspareunia.

Data about effectiveness of rehabilitation in pelvic floor dysfunction, so far reported, refer to general population. By now, there is a relevant number of studies which investigated the effectiveness of pelvic floor muscle training also in the specific population of pregnant and postpartum women, but almost exclusively looking at urinary incontinence. Moreover, pelvic floor muscle training was used as a preventive, therapeutic or mixed approach to incontinence, either during pregnancy or the postpartum period depending on the study, so data have to be examined in depth in this specific population.

A recent review on pregnancy- and postpartum-related pelvic floor disorders states that there is some evidence that, for women having their first baby, PFMT during pregnancy is effective in reducing incontinence up to 6 months after delivery, however this effect does not seem to persist after 1 year (preventive approach, providing PFMT to all continent women) [25]. More interesting, there is good evidence that PFMT is an appropriate treatment for women with persistent postpartum urinary incontinence (treatment approach, providing PFMT to incontinent women). The effect of a mixed prevention or treatment approach, providing PFMT to all women, continent or not, is less clear [26].

PFMT could have a long-term effect, as reported by Dumoulin, who showed benefits of physiotherapy for postpartum urinary incontinence still present 7 years after treatment [27], but this is not certain as other studies could not demonstrate any persistent effect of PFMT at 12 years [28].

Otherwise, evidence of PFMT effectiveness in the postpartum period in case of fecal incontinence is currently insufficient [25], although Glazener demonstrated a lower prevalence of FI in women after three sessions of training in PFMT after childbirth, showing a benefit that was not maintained at 12 years. Likewise, there are no data about PFMT in the treatment of pelvic organ prolapse, as the few studies (that could not demonstrate an advantage in providing PFMT) used a mixed approach to all women in the postpartum [29].

Another important key point in providing PFMT is the quality of intervention, as type of exercise, frequency, intensity and duration of training make the difference.

Training protocols can address from one to many follow-up sessions, which can be individual or group ones. Home training is currently associated with follow up by professionals, consisting of a different number of contractions/day.

15.3 What Are the Approaches to Pelvic Floor Dysfunctions After Childbirth?

A model for pelvic dysfunction care in pregnancy and postpartum should take into account on the one hand evidences for effectiveness of PFMT in this specific population, when available, otherwise in general population, and on the other hand sustainability by the National Health Service.

Strategies to deliver PFMT to women during pregnancy and in the postpartum period can vary from providing PFMT to all women, either symptomatic or not, as a preventive approach, to providing it only to symptomatic women as a specific treatment measure.

The first approach is probably not optimal while considering cost–benefit and sustainability of PFMT. A Cochrane review [25] states that "there is some evidence that for women having their first baby, PFMT can prevent urinary incontinence up to 6 months after delivery" but the cost of such an intervention in all primiparous women and the possible lack of long-term benefit discourage from this type of approach.

In fact, even the 5th International Consultation on Incontinence states: "it should be considered the cost–benefit of population-based approaches to health professional taught postpartum PFMT to all postpartum women regardless of their status" [18].

On the contrary the same Cochrane review concludes that there is support for the widespread recommendation that PFMT is an appropriate treatment for women with persistent postpartum urinary incontinence and that it is possible that the effects of PFMT might be greater with targeted approaches and in certain groups of women.

The identification of selection criteria for PFMT during pregnancy and after delivery is therefore a key point when developing a model of pelvic floor dysfunction care.

To this end the Italian Society of Urodynamics, continence, neurourology, and pelvic floor (SIUD) has developed a recording tool named "*SIUD postpartum pelvic dysfunctions card*" (SIUD PPD CARD) in order to provide a standardized evaluation system for epidemiological studies and to select women who could need conservative treatment in the postpartum period [30].

The SIUD PPD CARD moves from the idea that two different approaches in selecting women to refer to PFMT after delivery can be considered:

- A *risk factors approach*: selecting at hospital discharge women considered at risk of developing pelvic dysfunctions
- A *signs of damage approach*: selecting women who still have symptoms or signs of pelvic dysfunction at follow up in the postpartum period

The "*risk factor approach*" is used in more than one birth center, but it is not clear what risk factors are really to be considered, so selection criteria are not homogeneous. In the attempt to provide more uniformity to this approach a standardized tool (called "Perineal card") was developed in Italy, consisting of a checklist of risk factors resulting in a final risk score. On the basis of that score, women were addressed or not to a PFMT [31].

The risk factor approach has the advantage to provide to the birth center a simple way to select women who need more attention, due to an increased risk of developing pelvic floor dysfunctions. An analogous approach was proposed in a previous study by Chiarelli, even if this work took in account only two risk factors, forceps delivery or a vaginal delivery of a large baby >4,000 g [32].

Unfortunately, although some risk factors have been identified as significantly associated with the occurrence of pelvic floor trauma, at present there is no agreement about the combination and weight of factors that can influence the outcome in terms of urinary incontinence, prolapse, anal incontinence, pain and dyspareunia. The risk factors approach could imply missing women affected by pelvic dysfunctions who initially were considered at low risk and overtreating women considered at risk but with no pelvic dysfunctions. So this could be not the best way of selecting the group of women that most need a PFMT.

At the opposite, the "*signs of damage approach,*" adopted in other experiences as in the "Mothers without incontinence" Project, sponsored in 2003 by the Piedmont health authority [6], focuses attention on women who really have developed one or more dysfunctions as urinary or anal incontinence, prolapse, pain and dyspareunia. In this case the selection criteria were based on the presence at 2-month postpartum consultation of at least one among five symptoms or signs: urinary incontinence (if still persistent after 30 days after delivery), anal incontinence (if still persistent after 1 week after delivery); more than mild pain or dyspareunia still reported at the time of consultation; POP ≥2nd degree and perineal testing at digital palpations <2 in a 0–4 scale (AIPDA testing) [33].

The *signs of damage approach* has the advantage of selecting women who actually "have" pelvic floor dysfunction, narrowing patients' number in order to better address specific treatment resources. Moreover, it is quite common that women have their first postpartum consultation by a gynecologist who is not related to the delivery center. In this case, due to a lack of information about pregnancy and delivery risk factors, a "signs of damage approach" often represents the only way to deal with the problem.

15.3.1 The SIUD PPD Card

The aim of the Italian Society of Urodynamics Postpartum Pelvic Dysfunctions Card (SIUD PPD CARD) is to provide to all professionals a standard instrument to collect data for both kinds of approach: the *Risk Factor* and the S*igns of damage* approach. While the first one simply needs to collect data concerning pregnancy and delivery, the second approach is a little bit more complex, dealing with different anatomical compartments and functions. The guiding principles that led the birth of this tool were simplicity and, whenever possible, adoption of already validated instruments, in order to supply an instrument at the same time complete, valid and easy to use.

The result is a *"SIUD postpartum pelvic dysfunctions card"* composed of two different sections: a *"Delivery Card,"* collecting obstetrical data and potential *risk factors* and a *"Postpartum screening card"* collecting the *signs of damage*.

15.3.2 **Delivery Card** (Appendix A.1)

The *Delivery Card* includes the most significant obstetrical data and potential risk factors beside mother demographical data. It also takes into consideration urinary retention (if persistent 24 h after delivery) and preexisting or during pregnancy pelvic functional disorders.

This tool is intended to be completed by the clinical staff at the time of discharge from the birth center. Therefore, it should be available for the first puerperal consultation.

15.3.3 **Postpartum Screening Card** (Appendix A.2)

The "postpartum screening card" is intended to record the presence of pelvic dysfunctions after delivery. The card is composed of five sections: urinary incontinence, anal incontinence, pelvic organ prolapse, pain and dyspareunia and pelvic floor muscle dysfunction. Based on validated existing instruments every section includes a quantification system to provide an outcome measure for observational or interventional approaches. For each considered dysfunction an assessment tool is included in the card as follows:

1. Urinary incontinence: the ICI-q SF [8].
2. Anal incontinence: the so-called Wexner incontinence score [9].
3. Pelvic organ prolapse: POP-Q simplified staging system [10].
4. Pain and dyspareunia: visual analog system (VAS).
5. Pelvic floor muscle dysfunction: the Oxford modified grading system [11].

The card can be used as a simple recording tool but the Authors have also arbitrarily established a cut-off for every section (see Appendix A.2) that can be used as a selection parameter for management (counseling, lifestyle interventions, or rehabilitation according to the condition). In other words, when at least in one section the values exceed the cut-off, the woman is considered worthwhile of attention. In this way a population that need an intervention can be selected and have care for pelvic dysfunctions.

This tool is intended to be completed by the clinical staff at postpartum consultation.

Considering epidemiology, PFMT effectiveness and finally the insufficient public and professional awareness and availability of sanitary resources for management of pelvic dysfunctions, there is a need of more attention for the postpartum pelvic dysfunction problem. The SIUD PPD CARD is a standardized assessment tool that combines obstetrical data and signs and symptoms of pelvic floor dysfunction in the postpartum period. Providing a standardized evaluation and establishing criteria for selecting women who need care is a way to improve in future the management of women affected by postpartum pelvic dysfunction.

Appendix A.1

SIUD PPD CARD

The DELIVERY CARD

Surname……………………………………..Name……………(mother)
Delivery date …………/……/………………

	NUMBER / TEXT	YES	NO
Age *(mother)*			
Previous vaginal deliveries *(number)*			
BMI *(at delivery)*			
Dystocic labour *(type)*		yes	no
Shoulder dystocia		yes	no
Second stage of labour *(minutes)*			
Precipitous labour		yes	no
Induced labor (if "yes", specify the method: *oxytocine, prostaglandines, amniotomy/other*)		yes	no
If induced labor specify the clinical indication: *hypertensive disorders/gestational diabetes/post-term prolonged pregnancy/premature membrane rupture/other*			
Emergency caesarean section		yes	no
Elective caesarean section		yes	no
Episiotomy *(if "yes", specify if midline or mediolateral)*		yes	no
Vaginal-perineal tear *(0-4 scale as reported below)**		yes	no
Episiotomy complications *(infection, haematoma, tear, other)*			
Vacuum extraction delivery		yes	no
Forceps delivery		yes	no
Kristeller maneuver		yes	no
Epidural analgesia		yes	no
Cefalic circumference *(cm)*			
Fetal weight *(grams)*			
Twin birth *(number)*		yes	no
Labour position *(recumbent, squat, on all fours, on the side, into water, other)*			

Urinary retention after delivery (if persistent after 24 hours)	yes	no

Dysfunctions before delivery	Before pregnancy		During pregnancy	
Stress urinary incontinence	yes	no	yes	no
Urge urinary incontinence	yes	no	yes	no
Anal incontinence (flatus)	yes	no	yes	no
Anal incontinence (stool)	yes	no	yes	no
Dyspareunia	yes	no	yes	no

**Perineal-vaginal tear grading*

0 - Intact	No tissue separation at any site	
1 - First degree	Injury to skin only *(i.e. involving the fourchette, perineal skin and vaginal mucous membrane)*	
2 - Second degree	Injury to the perineum involving perineal muscles but not the anal sphincter	
3 - Third degree	Injury to perineum involving the anal sphincter complex	• 3a: Less than 50% of external anal sphincter thickness torn • 3b: More than 50% of external anal sphincter thickness torn • 3c: Both internal and external anal sphincter torn
4 -Fourth degree	Injury to perineum involving the anal sphincter complex (external and internal anal sphincter) and anal epithelium and /or rectal mucosa)	

Appendix A.2

SIUD PPD CARD

POSTPARTUM SCREENING CARD

1) URINARY INCONTINENCE

☐ YES ☐ NO

Type: ☐ stress ☐ urge ☐ mixed ☐ other

ICIQ-SF

(INTERNATIONAL CONSULTATION ON INCONTINENCE QUESTIONNAIRE SHORT FORM)

Thinking about how you have been, on average, over the past four weeks:

1. How often do you leak urine?*
   - ☐ 0 **never**
   - ☐ 1 **about once a week or less often**
   - ☐ 2 **two or three times a week**
   - ☐ 3 **about once a day**
   - ☐ 4 **several times a day**
   - ☐ 5 **all the time**

2. We would like to know how much urine you think leaks.
   How much urine do you usually leak (whether you wear protection or not)?
   - ☐ 0 **None**
   - ☐ 2 **A small amount**
   - ☐ 4 **A moderate amount**
   - ☐ 6 **A large amount**

3. Overall, how much does leaking urine interfere with your everyday life?
   Please ring a number between 0 (not at all) and 10 (a great deal)

   ☐ 0 ☐ 1 ☐ 2 ☐ 3 ☐ 4 ☐ 5 ☐ 6 ☐ 7 ☐ 8 ☐ 9 ☐ 10

☐ *tick the box if you leak urine more than once a month, less than once a week

CUT OFF

SCORE >=1

2) ANAL INCONTINENCE

Fecal incontinence	☐ yes	☐ no	
Flatus incontinence	☐ yes	☐ no	
Soiling	☐ yes	☐ no	
Type of incontinence	☐ passive	☐ urge	☐ mixed

WEXNER SCORE

Incontinence	**Never**	**Rarely** Less than 1/month	**Sometimes** More than 1/month Less than 1/week	**Usually** More than 1/week Less than 1/day	**Always** Once a day or more
Solid	0	1	2	3	4
Liquid	0	1	2	3	4
Gas	0	1	2	3	4
Wear pad	0	1	2	3	4
Lyfestyle altered	0	1	2	3	4

Total score ☐

CUT OFF

At least 1 of the following :

- **SCORE > 0 *(almost 1)*if solid or liquid incontinence**
- **SCORE > 1 *(almost 2)* if flatus incontinence**

3) PELVIC ORGAN PROLAPSE

Simplified POP-Q STAGING

STAGE 0	No prolapse demonstrated
STAGE 1	Most distal portion of the prolapse is more than 1 cm above the level of the hymen
STAGE 2	Most distal portion of the prolapse is 1 cm or less proximal to or distal to the plane of the hymen
STAGE 3	The most distal portion of the prolapse is more than 1 cm below the plane of the hymen.
STAGE 4	Complete eversion of the total length of the lower genital tract is demonstrated

Most distal portion is:

☐ anterior ☐ central ☐ posterior

CUT OFF
STAGE $\geq$ 2

4) PERINEAL PAIN AND DYSPAREUNIA

	YES	NO
1-Perineal pain		
2- If "yes", do you think it is a problem for you?		
3-Dyspareunia		
4- If "yes", do you think it is a problem for you?		
5- Resumption of sexual acitivity		
6- If "yes", how many weeks after delivery?		

PERINEAL PAIN

VISUAL ANALOG SCALE (0-10)

DYSPAREUNIA

VISUAL ANALOG SCALE (0-10)

MARINOFF dyspareunia scale

0- No dyspareunia
1- Intercourse is painful but the degree of discomfort does not prevent penetration
2- The pain prevents intercourse from taking place on most occasions
3-Pain results in total apareunia

REDUCED VAGINAL SENSITIVITY AT INTERCOURSE
(compared to pre-pregnancy sensitivity)

VISUAL ANALOG SCALE (0-10)

CUT OFF
If perineal pain or dyspareunia are a problem
(if answered "yes" to questions 2 or 4)

5) PELVIC FLOOR MUSCLE DYSFUNCTION

MODIFIED OXFORD GRADING

0 = nil (no discernibile muscle contraction)

1 = flicker (a flicker or pulsation is felt under the examiner's finger)

2 = weak (an increase in tension is detected without any discernible lift)

3 = moderate (muscle tension is further enhanced and characterized by lifting of the muscle belly and also elevation of the posterior vaginal wall; a grade 3 or stronger can be observed as an in-drawing of the perineum and anus)

4 = good (increased tension and a good contraction are present which are capable of elevating the posterior vaginal wall against resistence)

5 = strong (strong resistance can be applied to the elevation of the posterior vaginal wall; the examining finger is squeezed and drawn into the vagina)

Grade ☐

If asymmetria: left ☐

right ☐

CUT OFF

Grade $\leq$ 2

(even if one side only)

Summary: Selection Criteria for Management

Dysfunction	Evaluation tool	Cut off
UI	ICI q SF	>1
AI	Wexner score	>1 if solid or liquid and/or >2 if gas
POP	Simplified POP q staging	> or = 2
Pain/dyspareunia	VAS	If it is a problem for the woman
Pelvic floor	Oxford score	< or = 2

References

1. van Brummen HJ, Bruinse HW, van de Pol G et al (2006) Bothersome lower urinary tract symptoms 1 year after first delivery: prevalence and the effect of childbirth. BJU Int 98(1):89–95
2. Chang SR, Chen KH, Lin HH et al (2014) Association of mode of delivery with urinary incontinence and changes in urinary incontinence over the first year postpartum. Obstet Gynecol 123(3):568–577
3. Torrisi G, Minini G, Bernasconi F (2012) A prospective study of pelvic floor dysfunctions related to delivery. Eur J Obstet Gynecol Reprod Biol 160(1):110–115
4. Thom DH, Rortveit G (2010) Prevalence of postpartum urinary incontinence: a systematic review. Acta Obstet Gynecol Scand 89(12):1511–1522
5. Johannessen HH, Wibe A, Stordahl A et al (2014) Prevalence and predictors of anal incontinence during pregnancy and 1 year after delivery: a prospective cohort study. BJOG 121(3):269–279
6. Fritel X, Khoshnood B, Fauconnier A (2013) Specific obstetrical risk factors for urinary versus anal incontinence 4 years after first delivery. Prog Urol 23(11):911–916
7. King VG, Boyles SH, Worstell TR (2010) Using the Brink score to predict postpartum anal incontinence. Am J Obstet Gynecol 203(5):486
8. Glazener C, Elders A, Macarthur C (2013) Childbirth and prolapse: long-term associations with the symptoms and objective measurement of pelvic organ prolapse. BJOG 120(2): 161–168
9. O'Boyle AL, O'Boyle JD, Calhoun B et al (2005) Pelvic organ support in pregnancy and postpartum. Int Urogynecol J Pelvic Floor Dysfunct 16(1):69–72
10. Sze EH, Sherard GB 3rd, Dolezal JM et al (2002) Pregnancy, labor, delivery, and pelvic organ prolapse. Obstet Gynecol 100(5 Pt 1):981–986
11. Chen Y, Li FY, Lin X et al (2013) The recovery of pelvic organ support during the first year postpartum. BJOG 120(11):1430–1437
12. Handa VL, Nygaard I, Kenton K et al (2009) Pelvic organ support among primiparous women in the first year after childbirth. Int Urogynecol J Pelvic Floor Dysfunct 20(12):1407–1411
13. Tennfjord MK, Hilde G, Stær-Jensen J, Ellström Engh M et al (2014) Dyspareunia and pelvic floor muscle function before and during pregnancy and after childbirth. Int Urogynecol J 25(9):1227–1235
14. Serati M, Salvatore S, Khullar V et al (2008) Prospective study to assess risk factors for pelvic floor dysfunction after delivery. Acta Obstet Gynecol Scand 87(3):313–318
15. Connolly A, Thorp J, Pahel L (2005) Effects of pregnancy and childbirth on postpartum sexual function: a longitudinal prospective study. Int Urogynecol J Pelvic Floor Dysfunct 16:263–267
16. Tunn R, DeLancey JO, Howard D (1999) MR imaging of levator ani muscle recovery following vaginal delivery. Int Urogynecol J Pelvic Floor Dysfunct 10(5):300–307

17. Peschers UM, Schaer GN, DeLancey JO et al (1997) Levator ani function before and after childbirth. Br J Obstet Gynaecol 104(9):1004–1008
18. Abrams P, Cardozo L, Khoury S, Wein A (ed) (2012) Incontinence. 5th international consultation on incontinence, Paris
19. Braekken IH, Majida M, Engh ME (2010) Can pelvic floor muscle training reverse pelvic organ prolapse and reduce prolapse symptoms? An assessor-blinded, randomized, controlled trial. Am J Obstet Gynecol 203(2):170
20. Hagen S, Stark D, Glazener C (2014) Individualised pelvic floor muscle training in women with pelvic organ prolapse (POPPY): a multicentre randomised controlled trial. Lancet 383(9919):796–806
21. Norton C, Cody JD (2012) Biofeedback and/or sphincter exercises for the treatment of faecal incontinence in adults. Cochrane Database Syst Rev (7). doi:10.1002/14651858.CD002111.pub3
22. Montorsi F, Basson R, Adaikan G et al (eds) (2010) Sexual medicine: sexual dysfunctions in men and women. Health Publication Ltd, Paris
23. Bergeron S, Khalifé S, Glazer HI (2008) Surgical and behavioral treatments for vestibulodynia: two-and-one-half year follow-up and predictors of outcome. Obstet Gynecol 111(1):159–166
24. Glazer HI, Rodke G, Swencionis C (1995) Treatment of vulvar vestibulitis syndrome with electromyographic biofeedback of pelvic floor musculature. J Reprod Med 40(4):283–290
25. Boyle R, Hay-Smith EJC, Cody JD et al (2014) Pelvic floor muscle training for prevention and treatment of urinary and fecal incontinence in antenatal and postnatal women: a short version Cochrane Review. Neurourol Urodyn 33(3):269–276
26. Hilde G, Stær-Jensen J, Siafarikas F et al (2013) Postpartum pelvic floor muscle training and urinary incontinence: a randomized controlled trial. Obstet Gynecol 122(6):1231–1238
27. Dumoulin C, Martin C, Elliott V et al (2013) Randomized controlled trial of Physiotherapy for postpartum stress incontinence: 7-year follow-up. Neurourol Urodyn 32:449–454
28. Glazener CM, MacArthur C, Hagen S (2014) Twelve-year follow-up of conservative management of postnatal urinary and faecal incontinence and prolapse outcomes: randomised controlled trial. BJOG 121(1):112–120
29. Bø K, Hilde G, Stær-Jensen J, Siafarikas F et al (2015) Postpartum pelvic floor muscle training and pelvic organ prolapse-a randomized trial of primiparous women. Am J Obstet Gynecol 212(1):38.e1–7
30. Biroli A, Soligo M, Bernasconi F et al (2013) The "Italian Society of Urodynamics' (SIUD) delivery & pelvic dysfunctions card": an Italian language screening tool. Pelviperineology 32:81–85
31. Zanelli S, Minini GF, Gatti D (2002) Perineal care program (PCP): un progetto di tutela della salute perineale nelle varie fasi del percorso biologico della donna. Urogynaecologia Int J 1(Suppl 16):178–82
32. Chiarelli P, Cockburn J (2002) Promoting urinary continence in women after delivery: randomised controlled trial. BMJ 324(7348):1241
33. Biroli A, Castellino C, Bellora MG et al (2004) Post-partum pelvic floor dysfunctions: prevalence and management. Urodinamica 14:274–277

Clinical Cases 16

Arianna Bortolami

16.1 Introduction

The presence of symptoms related to pelvic floor dysfunction after delivery can result in a serious impairment of quality of life [1, 2] in a time in which, on the contrary, the woman, the couple and the family could enjoy a great happiness. Among these problems, the most frequently reported are bladder storage symptoms, such as urinary incontinence, and pelvic organ prolapse; while anal incontinence and/or faecal incontinence or dyspareunia are more rarely reported, we can suspect that the percentage of the latter two may be higher. In some cases, these symptoms undergo a spontaneous remission, whereas in other cases they remain with no or little change. The solution for these conditions may involve both conservative therapies, and drugs or surgical managements, depending on the condition. Evaluation and consideration of scientific evidences enable the appropriate management of these patients. It is also remarkable to emphasize the importance of health professionals who must help women to reveal these conditions, that are often hidden, and to promote care, also in relationship to long-term consequences.

16.2 Case 1: Silvia, Urinary Incontinence

1. *Symptoms and complaints reported*
   Silvia, 38 years, complains of urinary incontinence. She reveals that this symptom had already occurred after the first vaginal childbirth 3 years before, but had regressed spontaneously after about 1 month. It has come back during the second pregnancy; she gave birth 4 months earlier. The symptom occurred mainly during

A. Bortolami
Private Practitioner, Studio di Fisioterapia 3D, Via Roberto Marin 17 A, Padova 35122, Italy
e-mail: arianna.bortolami@gmail.com

D. Riva, G. Minini (eds.), *Childbirth-Related Pelvic Floor Dysfunction: Risk Factors, Prevention, Evaluation, and Treatment*,
DOI 10.1007/978-3-319-18197-4_16

sport activities, especially in the gym that the patient has begun recently, but that she stopped in frustration due to incontinence. The symptom occurs sometimes during coughing, sneezing and laughing. The patient is very worried, also for the desire of a third pregnancy.

2. *History*
   - Use of pads: daytime use, little size, 1/day
   - Nocturia: 1/2 vv/night. Absent during previous pregnancies
   - Pregnancies and births: two vaginal physiologic deliveries, the first 3 years before, with episiotomy, the second 4 months before
   - Regular menstrual cycle since 3 months
   - kg 62, mt 1.7,1 BMI 21.20
   - No other pathologies
   - No use of drugs
   - No surgery
3. *Physical examination*
   No significant urethral hypermobility. No signs of pelvic organ prolapse. The levator muscle contraction is present. Negative stress test.
4. *Instrumental diagnostics*
   URODYNAMIC INVESTIGATIONS
   Cystomanometry: Parameters of bladder storage are characterized by normal sensitivity, compliance and capacity (450 ml). Stable detrusor. Involuntary loss of urine with provocative manoeuvres (cough, hops) at 400 cc. Emptying the bladder with detrusor use of the catheter. Non-significant post-voiding residual (about 30 cc.).
5. *Presumptive diagnosis*: Stress urinary incontinence
6. *Treatment*
   The patient is directed to conservative treatment, specifically pelvic floor physical therapy and rehabilitation [3].
   PELVIC FLOOR PHYSICAL THERAPY AND REHABILITATION:
   A. *Functional Assessment*
      In addition to the above, the following points are highlighted:
      - Urinary loss in drops, sensitivity refers to the loss
      - Evolution of the onset of the disorder: worse
      - Relationship to other situations than those reported during urinary loss: none
      - Voiding frequency: every 1/2 h. Before pregnancies, the frequency was every 3/4 h
      - Use of preventive urination for about 4/5 vv / day
      - Reported "stop urine stream" performed several times at the suggestion, but stopped for failure in the execution
      - Hydration: 1.5 l reported
      - No urinary urgency
      - No symptoms related to bladder emptying phase
      - No cystitis
      - No anal or faecal incontinence
      - Reported occasional constipation (straining >5′)

B. *Physical Examination*

B1. VISUAL INSPECTION: Normally closed labia, length of the tendinous centre of the perineum 3 cm, intacted skin and mucous membranes and normal in colour and trophism. No evidence of anatomical changes. At the request of the voluntary contraction of the pelvic floor, the patient is able to perform it, even in the presence of biomechanical compensation to the hamstring and gluteal muscles. Negative stress test.

B2. MANUAL ASSESSMENT: Normal tone and trophism of the levator ani muscle. Parameters muscle bundles of the levator to the request for voluntary contraction (classification ICS / IUGA 2010) [4, 5]: weak force, weak tightness, normal fatigue, complete relaxation. At the request of straining, there is a good muscle relaxation. During cough, weak reflex contraction of the levator ani.

B3. PAPER ASSESSMENT

BLADDER DIARY: Administered for 5 days, including weekend. Daily frequency: 13. Night frequency: 1.5. Urgency: absent. Max voided volume: 200 ml. Hydration: 1,500 ml

TEST AND QUESTIONNAIRES:

King's Health Questionnaire: 59

ICIQ-SF: 3/2/4; IQOL: 88.

C. *Planning* [6]:

Therapeutic Goals: Improve muscle strength parameter, especially in relationship to reflex contraction during rises in intra-abdominal pressure [7]; in this way add sport activity in the absence of urinary leakage.

Techniques and Tools: Pelvic floor muscles therapeutic exercise, biofeedback (if necessary), bladder training, functional electrical stimulation, self-home training, behavioural therapy.

D. *Intervention:*

After awareness for pelvic floor, the importance of not urinating in a preventive way is immediately highlighted; the importance of avoiding straining during defecation is also stressed. After one session, the patient performs the selective contraction of pelvic floor muscles. Subsequently, muscle strength is emphasized and is used functional electrical stimulation, which the patient performs daily at home for about 2 months. At about 40 days from the beginning of the physical and rehabilitation therapy, the "knack" is learned, to be performed whenever the symptom occurs.

E. *Evaluation:*

After three sessions, the patient begins to report improvements. Then, after a short interval, she improves again to reach the condition of total dry; she needs to use "the knack".

7. *Results*: At the end of the pelvic floor physical therapy and rehabilitation, the patient is referred to a situation without involuntary loss of urine.

King's Health Questionnaire: 23

ICIQ-SF: 0,5/2/0; IQOL: 94

8. *Follow-Up*
   Six months after the end of pelvic floor physical therapy and rehabilitation, the results are maintained using the “knack” during significant increase in intra-abdominal pressure [8]. The patient is satisfied with the results.
   King’s Health Questionnaire: 25
   ICIQ-SF: 0,5/2/0; IQOL: 93

16.3 Case 2: Margherita, Dyspareunia

1. *Symptoms and complaints reported*
   Margherita, age 32, had a vaginal birth 6 months before (a male fetus weighing 3,200 kg), during which a third-degree laceration occurred. After 1 month, she tried to restore sexual activity, but with pain. Then she rarely tried again, but always having to stop the attempts of penetration due to severe pain and burning. For 2 months, she suspended every attempt. She declares that this symptom is becoming a serious personal and couple problem, and that it is worsening irremediably this period of her life, which was expected to be rather wonderful. She also reports that she was referred to another specialist, who suggested to wait for spontaneous recovery.
2. *History*
   No pain or other problems during sexual activity during the time before birth are reported, and this function is referred to as quite satisfactory. Regular cycle, now absent for breastfeeding. She does not report sense of weight, or vaginal and/or anal protrusion. Urinary incontinence or other symptoms related to bladder emptying are not present. No presence of symptoms related to the phase of bladder filling. Symptoms of abnormal rectal filling or empting not reported..
3. *Physical examination*
   Episiotomy at the left side, normal skin, reddened mucosa, especially in the lower portion of the vagina. At the request of voluntary muscle contraction, absence of recruitment of pelvic floor muscles.
   Swab test positive between 5 and 7, VAS 8/10. The introduction of the examiner’s finger, while tolerated, causes a burning sensation. Increased muscle tone at the left branch of the levator ani, normal on the right; hypotonus on both sides, particularly on the right. Absence of the request for voluntary contraction; at the request of straining, there is a partial relaxation of levator muscle.
4. *Diagnosis*: Dyspareunia and vulvar vestibulitis after delivery [9–12].
5. *Treatment*: Physiotherapy and pelvic floor rehabilitation are recommended [13–15]. Use of topical anti-inflammatory may be useful.
   PELVIC FLOOR PHYSICAL THERAPY AND REHABILITATION:
   A. *Functional Assessment*
      The previous history is confirmed.
   B. *Physical Examination*
      In addition to the above, these points are highlighted:
      - Important compensation with activation of the abdominal wall during the attempted voluntary contraction

- At the request of straining, there is the levator ani partial relaxation.

B3. PAPER ASSESSMENT

FSFI: 23 [16]

Mc Gill Pain Questionnaire: The pain appears like a needle hole, is sharp as a razor blade and propagates burning and torturing.

VAS 10 during the penetration attempts.

C. *Planning*

Therapeutic Goals: Reduce pain and burning on the vaginal vestibule, improve pelvic floor muscles relaxation, restore satisfactory sexual function

Techniques and Tools: Pelvic floor muscles therapeutic exercise, biofeedback (if necessary), manual therapy, non-drugs topic products, vaginal dilators, self-home training

D. *Intervention*

The initial phase of awareness and voluntary motor activity of the pelvic floor muscles is more complex for this patient (four dates). Then, priority is given to the use of muscle relaxation (Fig. 16.1). Subsequently, the use of manual therapy facilitates the recovery of this parameter's muscular and viscoelastic properties of the pelvic floor muscles. After that, vaginal dilators are used. The patient performs self-training at home on a daily basis, including the techniques already used in the therapeutic setting. Since the beginning of treatment, the use of non-drugs topical products is proposed.

6. *Results*

At 5 months since the beginning of pelvic floor physical therapy and rehabilitation, the patient reported the resumption of sexual activity that occurs without pain, but without the pleasure present before birth. Over the next 2 months, the patient improves sexual function and reported a satisfactory recovery.

FSFI: 63

7. *Follow-Up*

Four months after the end of physical therapy, the patient reported satisfaction with the maintenance of the results.

FSFI: 85

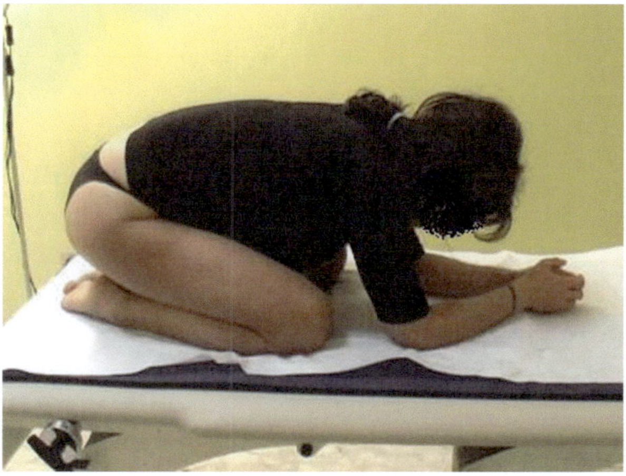

Fig. 16.1 Position used to relax and stretching pelvic floor muscles

16.4 Case 3: Anna, Rectocele (with the Courtesy of Vittorio Piloni)

1. *Symptoms, complaints reported, history, physical examination*
   ANNA, 49-year-old, weight 67 kg; height 167 cm, BMI 25.2, multiparous woman (three pregnancies with three vaginal births), currently in surgical menopause. *History* of vaginal hysterectomy in 2010 due to pelvic organ prolapse; surgery for urethral caruncle in 2014. First-degree ano-vaginal tear at first delivery without episiotomy. *Presenting symptoms* of difficult defecation, fractionated stools, becoming worse during the last year. Stool frequency: 2–3 times in the day, with frequent sensation of incomplete emptying. She can defecate without digitation. Urinary stress incontinence is complained. Large rectocele is noted at *physical examination.* Anal tonus is normal, and so are strength, endurance and relaxation. At vaginal inspection, hypotone, decreased contractile activity and endurance are appreciated.
2. *Instrumental diagnosis:*
   COLONSCOPY: negative
   MR DEFECOGRAPHY
   See Fig. 16.2a, b
3. *Diagnosis*
   Rectocele
4. *Treatment*
   Surgery has been proposed to the patient, who accepted.
5. *Results*
   One year after surgery, the patient reported great improvement during defecation and is satisfied with the result.

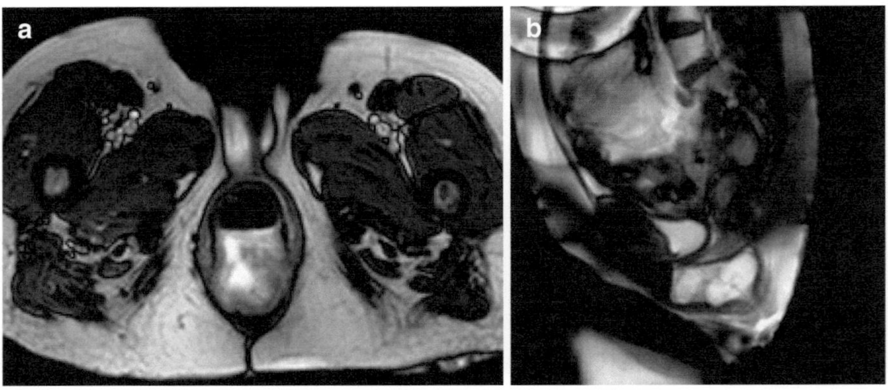

Fig. 16.2 (**a**) Axial image of the levator hiatus on straining, BFFE pulse sequence: large (>4 cm deep) rectocele projecting beyond the hymen; (**b**) midsagittal image taken during evacuation of rectal contrast (acoustic jelly) showing large rectocele due to displacement (Type 1) of pelvic organs

16.5 Case 4: Valeria, Obstructed Defecation (with the Courtesy of Vittorio Piloni)

1. *Symptoms, complaints reported, history, physical examination*
   A 55-year-old multiparous woman (weight, 65 kg; height 165 cm, BMI, 23.9) currently in menopause, with *history* of third-degree ano-vaginal tear at first delivery, development of utero-vaginal prolapse at 1 year from the fourth childbirth and subsequent surgical repair with combined hysterectomy and vaginoplasty 5 years later. *Presenting symptoms* include obstructed defecation syndrome since 2 years with recent worsening, sensation maintained but feeling of unsatisfactory evacuation and incomplete emptying, weight sensation and need for manual squeezing of the perineal region to complete the evacuation. Stool frequency: once every 2–3 days. Additional lower urinary tract (LUT) symptoms reported include the following: increased daily and nocturnal frequency, occasional urinary stress incontinence, hesitancy and need for abdominal straining to assist and complete voiding. Other general symptoms include back lumbar pain since 2 years. At *physical examination*, with no evidence of any wall bulging, a definite vaginal gaping is appreciated together with hypertonic external anal sphincter and puborectalis muscle, weak voluntary contractile activity of the pelvic floor musculature, reduced genital hiatus widening on Valsalva manoeuvre and paradoxical contraction of the levator ani (LA) muscle. More precisely, while a muscular hypotone and decreased contractile activity is appreciated in the right limb of the LA, a hypertone and normal relaxation is observed in the left limb.
2. *Instrumental diagnosis:*
   MANOMETRY

   Conclusions: Increased resting tone, insufficient increase in pressure at voluntary contraction. High-pressure zone length of 2.4 cm. RIRA elicited at 140 ml. Ampullary first sensation increased. Relaxation of the sphincter to distension of the rectum reduced with a paradoxical contraction during straining. Manometric framework compatible with obstructed defecation syndrome.

   MR DEFECOGRAPHY

   See Fig. 16.3a, b
3. *Diagnosis*
   Obstructed defecation syndrome linked to a paradoxical contraction of pelvic floor muscles
4. *Treatment*
   Conservative, pelvic floor physical therapy and rehabilitation
   PELVIC FLOOR PHYSICAL THERAPY AND REHABILITATION:
   E. *Functional Assessment*
      In addition to the above, we have highlighted:
      - Sometimes, with sensation for evacuation, she is not satisfied with it.
      - Sometimes she tries to defecate without sensation for evacuation.

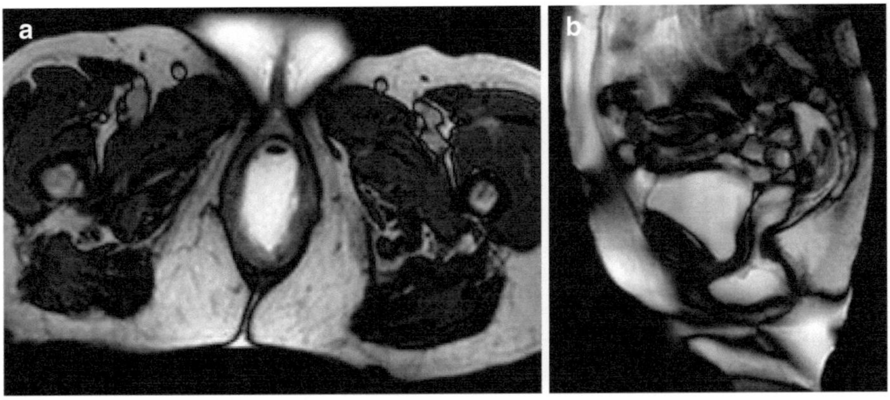

Fig. 16.3 (**a**) Axial image of the levator hiatus on straining, BFFE pulse sequence: large (>4 cm deep) rectocele projecting beyond the hymen indistinguishable from that of type I rectocele; (**b**) midsagittal image taken during evacuation showing protrusion of the anterior rectal wall and an asymmetric "sand glass" appearance of the ano-rectal junction (Type II rectocele) with persistent impression of the puborectalis muscle due to dyssynergic contraction of the levator ani muscle

F. *Physical Examination*

In addition to the above, we have highlighted:

- Negative stress test.

B3. PAPER ASSESSMENT

WEXNER CONSTIPATION SCORE: 15/30

SF-36: Physical Functioning 90/100; Role-Physical 25/100; Body Pain 84/100; General Health 20/100; Vitality 35/100; Social Role 37/100; Emotional Role 0/100; Mental Health 24/100.

G. *Planning*

Therapeutic Goals: Improve the coordination of puborectalis muscle during straining, decrease hypertonus of puborectalis muscle and external anal sphincter, normalize bowel habits

Techniques and Tools: Pelvic floor muscles therapeutic exercise, biofeedback, rectal balloon, manual therapy, behavioural therapy, bowel training, anal dilators [17–20]

INTERVENTION:

An explanation about functioning of pelvic floor muscles has been presented, especially of the posterior region. The patient has been instructed not to strain without sensation to defecate and to defecate when the same sensation is present. Therapeutic exercises to relax posterior pelvic floor muscles have been used; then biofeedback, rectal balloon, manual therapy permitted the right coordination of puborectalis muscle (2 months, 1 times a week). Anal dilators have been used for hypertone. The patient used the exercise and anal dilators every day at home.

5. *Results*

At the end of pelvic floor physical therapy and rehabilitation, the patient defecates once a day, almost every day; most of times she feels satisfactory evacuating and complete emptying. She very rarely needs a manual sustainment of the perineal region to assist the evacuation.

WEXNER CONSTIPATION SCORE: 5/30

SF-36: Physical Functioning 100/100; Role-Physical 75/100; Body Pain 100/100; General Health 86/100; Vitality 35/100; Social Role 75/100; Emotional Role 66/100; Mental Health 68/100.

6. *Follow-Up*

Six months after the end of physical therapy, the patient reported satisfaction with the maintenance of the results.

WEXNER CONSTIPATION SCORE: 4

SF-36: Physical Functioning 100/100; Role-Physical 73/100; Body Pain 100/100; General Health 88/100; Vitality 36/100; Social Role 75/100; Emotional Role 68/100; Mental Health 70/100.

References

1. van Delft K, Sultan A, Thakar R, Schwertner-Tiepelmann N, Kluivers K (2014) The relationship between postpartum levator ani muscle avulsion and signs and symptoms of pelvic floor dysfunction. BJOG 121(9):1164–1172. doi:10.1111/1471-0528.12666, Epub 2014 Feb 19
2. Schwertner-Tiepelmann N, Thakar R, Sultan AH, Tunn R (2012) Obstetric levator ani muscle injuries: current status. Ultrasound Obstet Gynecol 39(4):372–383
3. Herschorn S, Hosker G, Kelleher C, Koelbl H, Khoury S, Madoff R, Milsom I, Moore K, Newman D, Nitti V, Norton C, Nygaard I, Payne C, Smith A, Staskin D, Tekgul S, Thuroff J, Tubaro A, Vodusek D, Wein A, Wyndaele JJ, Members of Committees; Fourth International Consultation on Incontinence (2010) Fourth International Consultation on Incontinence Recommendations of the International Scientific Committee: evaluation and treatment of urinary incontinence, pelvic organ prolapse, and fecal incontinence. Neurourol Urodyn 29:213–240
4. Haylen BT, de Ridder D, Freeman RM, Swift SE, Berghmans B, Lee J, Monga A, Petri E, Rizk DE, Sand PK, Schaer GN (2010) An International Urogynecological Association (IUGA)/International Continence Society (ICS) joint report on the terminology for female pelvic floor dysfunction. Int Urogynecol J 21:5–26
5. Messelink B, Benson T, Berghmans B, Bø K, Corcos J, Fowler C, Laycock J, Lim PH, van Lunsen R, á Nijeholt GL, Pemberton J, Wang A, Watier A, Van Kerrebroeck P (2005) Standardization of terminology of pelvic floor muscle function and dysfunction: report From the Pelvic Floor Clinical Assessment Group of the International Continence Society. Neurourol Urodyn 24:374–380
6. Hay-Smith EJ, Herderschee R, Dumoulin C, Herbison GP (2011) Comparisons of approaches to pelvic floor muscle training for urinary incontinence in women. Cochrane Database Syst Rev (12):CD009508
7. Miller JM, Ashton-Miller JA, DeLancey JO (1998) A pelvic muscle precontraction can reduce cough-related urine loss in selected women with mild SUI. J Am Geriatr Soc 46(7):870–874
8. McLean L, Varette K, Gentilcore-Saulnier E, Harvey MA, Baker K, Sauerbrei E (2013) Pelvic floor muscle training in women with stress urinary incontinence causes hypertrophy of the urethral sphincters and reduces bladder neck mobility during coughing. Neurourol Urodyn 32(8):1096–1102
9. Basson R, Berman J, Burnett A, Derogatis L, Ferguson D, Fourcroy J, Goldstein I, Graziottin A, Heiman J, Laan E, Leiblum S, Padma-Nathan H, Rosen R, Segraves K, Segraves RT, Shabsigh R, Sipski M, Wagner G, Whipple B (2000) Report of the international consensus development conference on female sexual dysfunction: definitions and classifications. J Urol 163:888–893

10. Fashokun TB, Harvie HS, Schimpf MO, Olivera CK, Epstein LB, Jean-Michel M, Rooney KE, Balgobin S, Ibeanu OA, Gala RB, Rogers RG, Society of Gynecologic Surgeons' Fellows' Pelvic Research Network (2013) Sexual activity and function in women with and without pelvic floor disorders. Int Urogynecol J 24:91–97
11. Handa VL, Cundiff G, Chang HH, Helzlsouer KJ (2008) Female sexual function and pelvic floor disorders. Obstet Gynecol 111:1045–1052
12. Lukacz ES, Whitcomb EL, Lawrence JM, Nager CW, Contreras R, Luber KM (2007) Are sexual activity and satisfaction affected by pelvic floor disorders? Analysis of a community-based survey. Am J Obstet Gynecol 197:88.e1–6
13. Rosembaum TY (2005) Physiotherapy treatment of sexual pain disorders. J Sex Marital Ther 31:329–340
14. Rosenbaum TY, Owens A (2008) The role of pelvic floor physical therapy in the treatment of pelvic and genital pain-related sexual dysfunction (CME). J Sex Med 5:513–523
15. Rosenbaum TY (2007) Pelvic floor involvement in male and female sexual dysfunction and the role of pelvic floor rehabilitation in treatment: a literature review. J Sex Med 4:4–13
16. Filocamo MT, Serati M, Li Marzi V, Costantini E, Milanesi M, Pietropaolo A, Polledro P, Gentile B, Maruccia S, Fornia S, Lauri I, Alei R, Arcangeli P, Sighinolfi MC, Manassero F, Andretta E, Palazzetti A, Bertelli E, Del Popolo G, Villari D (2014) The Female Sexual Function Index (FSFI): linguistic validation of the Italian version. J Sex Med 11:447–453
17. Chiarelli P (2008) Systematic review: the management of constipation using physical therapies including biofeedback. Aust NZ Continence J 14(1):6–7, 9–11, 13
18. Chiarioni G, Hevmen S, Whiethead WE (2006) Biofeedback therapy for dyssynergic defecation. World J Gastroenterol 12(44):7069–7074
19. Heymen S, Wexner SD, Vickers D, Nougueras JJ, Weiss EG, Pirakarsky AJ (1999) Prospective, randomized trial comparing four biofeedback techniques for patients with constipation. Dis Colon Rectum 42(11):1388–1393
20. Chiarioni G, Whitehead WE, Pezza V, Morelli A, Bassotti G (2006) Biofeedback is superior to laxatives for normal transit constipation due to pelvic floor dyssynergia. Gastroenterology 130(3):657–664

Index

A
Action potential, propagation, 84–86
American Medical Systems (AMS) score system, 146
Anal canal, 51, 52, 54–57, 59, 61, 63
  dilators, 192
  incontinence (AI), 105, 106, 109–111, 115, 117, 126, 130, 171–173, 175, 176
  manometry, 148, 150
  rhabdosphincters, 9–10
  sphincter repair, 25, 31
  sphincters, 6–7
Anorectal dysfunction, 158
  function, 13
  junction, 54, 56
Artificial blue stool, 150

B
Balloon rectal test, 148–149
Behaviour treatment, 187, 192
Bio-feedback, 187, 189
Birth positions, 123
Bony pelvis, 2–3
Bowel symptoms, 44–45

C
Cesarean section, 136, 139
Childbirth, 135–140
  trauma, 130
Conservative treatment, 186
Constipation, 14
Continence reflex, 10

D
Delayed pushing, 120, 124, 125, 127
Delivery, 135–139
  card, 175, 176
Differential amplifiers, 86
Directed pushing, 124
3-D TPUS. *See* Three-dimensional transperineal ultrasonography (3-D TPUS)
Dynamic graciloplasty, 153
Dyspareunia, 102, 105, 108, 112, 172, 173, 175, 176
  after delivery, 185, 188–189

E
Electrical stimulation, 187
Electrode array, 86–88, 93
Electromyography (EMG), 147, 150, 156
  anal sphincter, 83, 84, 87–90, 92–94
Electronic (e-PAQ-PF), 42
Endoanal ultrasonography, 51, 54–57
Endopelvic fascia, 2, 16–21
Endovaginal ultrasonography, 51, 53–54
End-to-end technique, 151, 152
Epidural analgesia, 120, 124–126
EPIQ, 42
Episiotomy, 105–112, 117, 119–123, 125, 126, 128
  incontinence, 84, 93–96
  mediolateral, 84, 87, 89–94
  prevalence of, 94, 95
Etiology, 13, 14, 57, 147

D. Riva, G. Minini (eds.), *Childbirth-Related Pelvic Floor Dysfunction: Risk Factors, Prevention, Evaluation, and Treatment*,
DOI 10.1007/978-3-319-18197-4

External anal sphincter muscle (EAS), 4–6, 12, 13, 20, 51, 58, 59, 62
denervation, 83, 89–91, 93, 94
electromyography, 84, 94–96
innervation zones, 83, 89–92
tears, 83, 91, 93–95

F
Fascial support system, 20–21
Fecal incontinence, 13, 14, 51
prevalence of, 94, 95
social and economic costs, 94
Forceps delivery, 126, 130

G
Genital prolapse, 135–139
Guarding reflex, 10

H
Hands off Approach, 121
Hands on Approach, 120
History, 41–43

I
IFIP. *See* Integrated Fusion Imaging Protocol (IFIP)
Innervation zone (IZ)
anal sphincter, 83, 84, 87–90, 92–94
distribution of, 88, 91, 92
Integrated Fusion Imaging Protocol (IFIP), 70, 78–81
Internal anal sphincter (IAS), 6, 7, 13, 22, 51
Intersphincteric space, 57, 60
Intra-anal probes, 84
Intrapartum risk factors, 25, 26, 28
Italian Society of Urodynamics Postpartum Pelvic Dysfunctions Card (SIUD PPD CARD), 174–176

K
Kegel exercises, 118
Kinesitherapy, 130

L
Levator ani, 51, 53, 55, 60–62
avulsion, 112
innervation damage, 12–14
muscle, 137
Levator hiatus, 53, 55
Life style
intervention, 185, 188
recommendations, 116
Longitudinal muscle, 57
Lubrication disorders, 103

M
Magnetic resonance imaging (MRI), 69–81
Manual therapy, 189, 192
Mechanism of labour, 36, 38
Medical therapy, 151
Micturition, 116, 128, 129
dysfunction, 158
Motoneurons, 87
Motor control, 156
Motor unit (MU)
action potential (MUAP), 84–88
MRI. *See* Magnetic resonance imaging (MRI)

N
Neuroaprassia. *See* Sensory-motor disorders
Neuromuscular junction, 83–86
Neurosacral modulation, 151, 153
Neuro-urologic examination, 49

O
Obstetrical injuries, 119
anal sphincter injuries (OASIS), 29, 32, 106, 108, 109
lesions, 83
Obstructed defecation, 51
Occipito-posterior position, 127
Operative vaginal delivery, 109, 112
Overactive pelvic floor (OAPF), 158
Overlapping technique, 151, 152

P
Pad test, 43–45
Pain, 115, 117, 125–129
Pelvic and perineal pain, 158
Pelvic diaphragm, 4–6, 16, 18, 19
dysfunctions, 131
floor, 35–38, 115–119, 126, 127, 130
denervation, 109, 111, 112
disorders, 51–64
dysfunctions, 136, 138, 171–183
muscles, 187–189, 191, 192
muscles: strength evaluation, 49
muscles: therapeutic exercise, 187, 189, 192
muscles: therapy (PFMT), 151, 156

muscles: training, 118–119, 126
during vaginal birth, 28, 31
Pelvic organ prolapse (POP), 51, 115, 165–168, 172, 173, 176, 185, 186, 190
Perineal body, 54, 62–64
care, 115–131
damage, 105
hygiene, 128
lacerations, 25, 26
massage, 112, 117, 125, 126
pain, 105, 108
tears, 106
trauma, 115–117, 119–121, 124, 126–128, 130
PFMT in postnatal women, 130
Physical therapy and rehabilitation, 186–189, 191, 192
Physiotherapy, 155–162
POPQ-system, 46
Postnatal care, 128
Post-partum, 129, 136, 138–140
screening card, 175, 176
Postural balance, 156–157
disorders, 158
Post-void residual urine (PVR), 47–48
Pregnancy, 165, 167–168
Prevention, 138–139
Prolapse symptoms, 44
Prolonged second stage, 119, 125
Psychology, 104
Puboanalis muscle, 57
Puborectalis muscle, 53, 84, 88, 93
Pudendal nerve injuries, 109, 111
neuralgia, 158
terminal motor latency (PNTML), 145, 148
Puerperium, 129

Q
Q-tip test, 48
Questionnaires, 42, 45

R
Rectal balloon, 192
Rehabilitation treatment, 159–162
Risk factors, 116–117, 136–138
Ritgen's manoeuvre, 120, 121

S
Screening, 129
Second stage of labor, 119, 120, 122–126, 131
Sensory-motor disorders, 157
Sexual activity, 129
arousal, 101, 103
desire, 101, 103
dysfunctions, 101, 103, 104, 158
function, 167
intercourse, resumption, 102, 104
satisfaction, 102, 103
symptoms, 45
SIUD PPD CARD. *See* Italian Society of Urodynamics Postpartum Pelvic Dysfunctions Card (SIUD PPD CARD)
Solid sphere test, 149, 150
Sphincter capacity, 157
Standardization of episiotomies, 107
Stress test, 48, 49
Suturing techniques, 128

T
Three-dimensional ultrasonography, 51, 52, 54, 58, 62
Transanal ultrasonography, 147
Transperineal ultrasonography, 51, 52
Transvaginal ultrasound, 130
Transverse perinei muscle, 56, 62, 63

U
Urethra, , 4, 7, 12, 15–22
Urethral rhabdosphincters, 6, 10, 11
Urinary continence, 14–17
incontinence (UI), 115, 118, 136–139, 165–168, 171–176, 185, 186, 188
symptoms, 42–43
Urogenital diaphragm, 6, 15–17, 20
hiatus, 130
Uterosacral ligament, 64

V
Vaginal childbirth, 115, 119
delivery, 35, 36, 69–81
dilators, 189
Voiding diary, 41, 43–45

W
Warm compresses, 125
Water immersion, 125
Wexner score system, 146

MIX
Papier aus verantwortungsvollen Quellen
Paper from responsible sources
FSC® C105338

If you have any concerns about our products,
you can contact us on
ProductSafety@springernature.com

In case Publisher is established outside the EU,
the EU authorized representative is:
Springer Nature Customer Service Center GmbH
Europaplatz 3, 69115 Heidelberg, Germany

Printed by Libri Plureos GmbH
in Hamburg, Germany